Appalachian Nursing

Contributions to Southern Appalachian Studies

1. *Memoirs of Grassy Creek: Growing Up in the Mountains on the Virginia–North Carolina Line.* Zetta Barker Hamby. 1998
2. *The Pond Mountain Chronicle: Self-Portrait of a Southern Appalachian Community.* Edited by Leland R. Cooper and Mary Lee Cooper. 1998
3. *Traditional Musicians of the Central Blue Ridge: Old Time, Early Country, Folk and Bluegrass Label Recording Artists, with Discographies.* Marty McGee. 2000
4. *W.R. Trivett, Appalachian Pictureman: Photographs of a Bygone Time.* Ralph E. Lentz II. 2001
5. *The People of the New River: Oral Histories from the Ashe, Alleghany and Watauga Counties of North Carolina.* Edited by Leland R. Cooper and Mary Lee Cooper. 2001
6. *John Fox, Jr., Appalachian Author.* Bill York. 2003
7. *The Thistle and the Brier: Historical Links and Cultural Parallels Between Scotland and Appalachia.* Richard Blaustein. 2003
8. *Tales from Sacred Wind: Coming of Age in Appalachia. The Cratis Williams Chronicles.* Cratis D. Williams. Edited by David Cratis Williams and Patricia D. Beaver. 2003
9. *Willard Gayheart, Appalachian Artist.* Willard Gayheart and Donia S. Eley. 2003
10. *The Forest City Lynching of 1900: Populism, Racism, and White Supremacy in Rutherford County, North Carolina.* J. Timothy Cole. 2003
11. *The Brevard Rosenwald School: Black Education and Community Building in a Southern Appalachian Town, 1920–1966.* Betty J. Reed. 2004
12. *The Bristol Sessions: Writings About the Big Bang of Country Music.* Edited by Charles K. Wolfe and Ted Olson. 2005
13. *Community and Change in the North Carolina Mountains: Oral Histories and Profiles of People from Western Watauga County.* Compiled by Nannie Greene and Catherine Stokes Sheppard. 2006
14. *Ashe County: A History; A New Edition.* Arthur Lloyd Fletcher. 2009 [2006]
15. *The New River Controversy; A New Edition.* Thomas J. Schoenbaum. Epilogue by R. Seth Woodard. 2007
16. *The Blue Ridge Parkway by Foot: A Park Ranger's Memoir.* Tim Pegram. 2007
17. *James Still: Critical Essays on the Dean of Appalachian Literature.* Edited by Ted Olson and Kathy H. Olson. 2008
18. *Owsley County, Kentucky, and the Perpetuation of Poverty.* John R. Burch, Jr. 2008
19. *Asheville: A History.* Nan K. Chase. 2007
20. *Southern Appalachian Poetry: An Anthology of Works by 37 Poets.* Edited by Marita Garin. 2008
21. *Ball, Bat and Bitumen: A History of Coalfield Baseball in the Appalachian South.* L.M. Sutter. 2009
22. *The Frontier Nursing Service: America's First Rural Nurse-Midwife Service and School.* Marie Bartlett. 2009
23. *James Still in Interviews, Oral Histories and Memoirs.* Edited by Ted Olson. 2009

24. *The Millstone Quarries of Powell County, Kentucky.* Charles D. Hockensmith. 2009

25. *The Bibliography of Appalachia: More Than 4,700 Books, Articles, Monographs and Dissertations, Topically Arranged and Indexed.* Compiled by John R. Burch, Jr. 2009

26. *Appalachian Children's Literature: An Annotated Bibliography.* Compiled by Roberta Teague Herrin and Sheila Quinn Oliver. 2010

27. *Southern Appalachian Storytellers: Interviews with Sixteen Keepers of the Oral Tradition.* Edited by Saundra Gerrell Kelley. 2010

28. *Southern West Virginia and the Struggle for Modernity.* Christopher Dorsey. 2011

29. *George Scarbrough, Appalachian Poet: A Biographical and Literary Study with Unpublished Writings.* Randy Mackin. 2011

30. *The Water-Powered Mills of Floyd County, Virginia: Illustrated Histories, 1770–2010.* Franklin F. Webb and Ricky L. Cox. 2012

31. *School Segregation in Western North Carolina: A History, 1860s–1970s.* Betty Jamerson Reed. 2011

32. *The Ravenscroft School in Asheville: A History of the Institution and Its People and Buildings.* Dale Wayne Slusser. 2014

33. *The Ore Knob Mine Murders: The Crimes, the Investigation and the Trials.* Rose M. Haynes. 2013

34. *New Art of Willard Gayheart.* Willard Gayheart and Donia S. Eley. 2014

35. *Public Health in Appalachia: Essays from the Clinic and the Field.* Edited by Wendy Welch. 2014

36. *The Rhetoric of Appalachian Identity.* Todd Snyder. 2014

37. *African American and Cherokee Nurses in Appalachia: A History, 1900–1965.* Phoebe Ann Pollitt. 2016

38. *A Hospital for Ashe County: Four Generations of Appalachian Community Health Care.* Janet C. Pittard. 2016

39. *Dwight Diller: West Virginia Mountain Musician.* Lewis M. Stern. 2016

40. *The Brown Mountain Lights: History, Science and Human Nature Explain an Appalachian Mystery.* Wade Edward Speer. 2017

41. *Richard L. Davis and the Color Line in Ohio Coal: A Hocking Valley Mine Labor Organizer, 1862–1900.* Frans H. Doppen. 2016

42. *The Silent Appalachian: Wordless Mountaineers in Fiction, Film and Television.* Vicki Sigmon Collins. 2017

43. *The Trees of Ashe County, North Carolina.* Doug Munroe. 2017

44. *Melungeon Portraits: Exploring Kinship and Identity.* Tamara L. Stachowicz. 2018

45. *Always Been a Rambler: G.B. Grayson and Henry Whitter, Country Music Pioneers of Southern Appalachia.* Josh Beckworth. 2018

46. *Tommy Thompson: New-Timey String Band Musician.* Lewis M. Stern. 2019

47. *Appalachian Fiddler Albert Hash: The Last Leaf on the Tree.* Malcolm L. Smith with Edwin Lacy. 2020

48. *Junaluska: Oral Histories of a Black Appalachian Community.* Edited by Susan E. Keefe with the Junaluska Heritage Association. 2020

49. *Boone Before Boone: The Archaeological Record of Northwestern North Carolina Through 1769.* Tom Whyte. 2020

50. *From the Front Lines of the Appalachian Addiction Crisis: Healthcare Providers Discuss Opioids, Meth and Recovery.* Edited by Wendy Welch. 2020

51. *Writers by the River: Reflections on 40+ Years of the Highland Summer Conference.* Edited by Donia S. Eley and Grace Toney Edwards. 2021

52. *Wayne Howard: Old Time Music, the Hammons Family and Mountain Lore.* Lewis M. Stern. 2021

53. *Lost Cove, North Carolina: Portrait of a Vanished Appalachian Community, 1864–1957* Christy A. Smith. 2022

54. *LeConte Lodge: A Centennial History of a Smoky Mountain Landmark.* Tom Layton and Mike Hembree. 2024

55. *D.D. Dougherty, Lillie Dougherty and the Early Years of Appalachian State.* Doris Perry Stam. 2024

56. *Appalachian Nursing: A History, 1890–1960.* Sharon Loury. 2025

Appalachian Nursing
A History, 1890–1960

SHARON LOURY

CONTRIBUTIONS TO
SOUTHERN APPALACHIAN STUDIES, 56

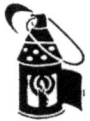

McFarland & Company, Inc., Publishers
Jefferson, North Carolina

ISBN (print) 978-1-4766-7541-1
ISBN (ebook) 978-1-4766-5494-2

Library of Congress cataloging data are available

Library of Congress Control Number 2025016234

© 2025 Sharon Loury. All rights reserved

No part of this book may be reproduced or transmitted in any form or by any means, electronic or mechanical, including photocopying or recording, or by any information storage and retrieval system, without permission in writing from the publisher.

Front cover images: Mary Rankin, teacher/nurse on horseback: home visit to a family in Vardy, Tennessee, c. 1920; Presbyterian Home Mission (lantern slide), (author's collection). Background: Blue Ridge Mountains © Jon Bilous/Shutterstock.

Printed in the United States of America

*McFarland & Company, Inc., Publishers
Box 611, Jefferson, North Carolina 28640
www.mcfarlandpub.com*

Acknowledgments

The author would like to thank the following individuals:

Sharon Bigger, RN, PhD—former East Tennessee State University PhD student (literature searches, interviews, annotated bibliography, collation of data/statistics)

Linda Cabage, RN, MSN, PhD candidate—East Tennessee State University PhD student (literature searches, annotated bibliography, Red Bird Mission visit with interviews)

Jane Harris, RN (retired)—Tennessee (coordination of a comprehensive exploration and documentation of the American Red Cross historical collections, documents, written materials, and photographs; a sincere thank you likewise goes to the American Red Cross nurses and staff who provided access to Jane for searches and assistance with collecting American Red Cross documents and written materials not available in archives or to the general public)

Evelyn Price Jones, RN (retired)—Jefferson, North Carolina (nurse who was educated and practiced in the Appalachian region prior to 1960 [personal conversation/accounts and photographs])

Agnes Lowe, RN (retired)—Johnson City, Tennessee (nurse who was educated and practiced in the Appalachian region prior to 1960 [personal conversation/accounts and photographs])

Billie McNamara, PhD candidate—Massachusetts (literature and archive searches, access to archived materials and documentation of Knoxville General Hospital School of Nursing's written materials, documents, and photographs)

Linda Simpson, RN, PhD—former East Tennessee State University PhD student (oral history of Trudy Fann)

Acknowledgments

A special thank you to:

Phoebe Pollitt, PhD, RN (retired associate professor of nursing, Appalachian State University, and nursing history author), for her prompting to write this book, introduction to the publishing team at McFarland, and support along the way

Martha Whaley (retired College of Medicine history of medicine librarian/services coordinator, East Tennessee State University) for access to library and museum materials, documents, photographs and archived holdings not available to the public and gift of the original NLNE series "List of Schools of Nurses Meeting Minimum Requirements Set by Law"

This book is a tribute to the memory of Dr. Barbara Brodie, PhD, RN (1935–2023), professor emerita, University of Virginia. Dr. Brodie was an eminent nurse historian, an educator, a mentor, a supporter, and the impetus for my journey into the heritage of nursing when I was a PhD student in the School of Nursing at the University of Virginia. I still remember Dr. Brodie's powerful remarks when I first met with her as a new student about to take her "History of Healthcare" course. I was trying to make a good impression and told her I was looking forward to her course and learning more about Florence Nightingale. Dr. Brodie looked at me, straightened up, and stated that while Florence Nightingale was renowned for her commendable work, there were many American nurses during those early decades who made significant contributions to the profession of nursing and nursing education in the United States.

Dr. Brodie was right.

Table of Contents

Acknowledgments — vii
Preface — 1
Introduction — 3

I. Geographic Setting and Early Healthcare — 7
II. The Evolution of Nursing Education and Professional Nursing — 24
III. Early Nursing Practice — 74

Conclusion — 173
References — 175
Index — 189

Preface

What originally started out as a single project in collaboration with a historian working on the history of a school of nursing in Knoxville, Tennessee, evolved into a larger regional historical study as new information emerged, suggesting that nursing throughout the core of the Appalachian region was not limited to one school, one role, one state or setting, but was part of a larger picture of healthcare within the entire region.

This particular history covers nursing education, hospitals, training schools, nurses, and their practice across the core of Appalachia from 1890 to 1960. A cross section of specific hospitals, training schools, and practice sites has been provided to illustrate the evolution of nursing throughout this region. Also included is historical background of the region and medicine, central to understanding the development of professional nursing in the region.

The book is organized into three main thematic chapters with related subtopics. In order to provide context and perspective for the reader, foundational information not necessarily exclusive or linked to Appalachia has also been provided.

Introduction

This history focuses on the evolution of nursing practice, nurses, nurses' education, and nurses' contributions to the health and well-being of those living in the core of Appalachia from 1890 to 1960. Historical research was conducted through the lens of sociopolitical and economic factors in the core of Appalachia within the context of medicine, hospitals, and associated organizations during this period that ultimately impacted the health of the regional population. Historical accounts of nursing in the United States have been well documented in numerous publications; however, the focus has been limited to large cities, or specific states, settings and groups, or general histories that span the entire United States. Except for a few group- and setting-specific accounts of nurses in Appalachia (Breckinridge, 1952; Cockerham & Keeling, 2012; Kirchgessner, 2000; Pollitt, 2014), the regional story of Appalachian nursing has not been told. Missing is the overall narrative of early nursing across the region in the context of the social and economic forces that shaped the culture of Appalachia.

Unknown to most, nurses in Appalachia played a significant role in the early healthcare of the population within the region and beyond, including the military and American Red Cross. The story of these nurses has not been recognized or documented as a regional entity but shared as separate, unconnected pieces of local history. Local accounts indicate the nurses who practiced in this region were resilient, dedicated, and innovative. They persevered, working through harsh and adverse conditions common to the rugged, rural, and isolated mountain communities. It was not uncommon for nurses to travel on horseback or on foot to reach residents in need of care in remote areas with few physicians or access to healthcare resources. Under austere conditions, the nurses were autonomous and innovative in addressing the needs of their patients. In many cases, they were surrogates for the physician,

Introduction

providing care beyond normal nursing practice. These dedicated nurses, together with physicians and healthcare organizations, helped shape professional healthcare in the Appalachian region.

Appalachia is a large, diverse area (spanning more than 1,000 miles, trailing along the Appalachian Mountains of the United States) and includes 13 states from northern Mississippi to southern New York. Nuances of social, cultural, and economic factors, as well as commonalities, trends, and traditions shared by community residents, exist within the subregions of Appalachia. The specific focus for this book centers on the core of Appalachia, a subregion of Central and Southern Appalachia designated and described by John Alexander Williams, a scholar of Appalachia (2002). Williams spent years researching this region and identified 165 counties among the states of Virginia, West Virginia, Tennessee, North Carolina, Kentucky, and Georgia that shared cultural, geographic, socioeconomic, and political similarities. These similarities played a significant role in the region's early healthcare, particularly regarding the cultural and sociopolitical impact on its residents.

A history of nursing in a single state may not necessarily capture the full essence of nursing within the core of Appalachia. Many nurses who were born in the region came from families with generational roots in Appalachia and inadequate financial resources. Prior to the late nineteenth century, some had never traveled outside the region and were limited in their ability to attend a professional nurses' training school, because such schools typically did not exist in the core of Appalachia. During this period, anyone who aspired to become a nurse would have to attend a training school in cities outside the Appalachian core, far from home. It wasn't until the very late 1890s that the first Nightingale-based training schools in the region began to emerge.

The lack of access to professional nursing education, however, did not preclude the practice of healthcare within the Appalachian region during the eighteenth and nineteenth centuries. Sources of early healing included lay healers, local Native Americans, granny midwives, and untrained physicians who had been practicing in the region since the very early 1800s. There were few (if any) professionally trained physicians available to care for the entire population, especially those communities in the more remote and isolated areas of Appalachia, where it could sometimes take days of travel over poor roads and rugged

Introduction

mountain terrain to reach a doctor's office or hospital. During that time, many community residents relied on family members and traditional healers to provide their healthcare. To this day, some residents may still rely on early healing remedies and practices.

The focus of research for this book has not been tethered or limited to one specific state or setting in Appalachia but spans the entire core of the Appalachian region. Primary sources; archived documents; historical archives; oral histories; family histories; interviews; written memoirs; letters; journals; newspaper accounts; autobiographies; and histories of training schools, organizations, and communities have been examined, analyzed, and synthesized in order to provide a documented account of nursing's evolution, role, and contributions to healthcare in the Appalachian region and beyond.

In the analysis of multiple sources and materials, several significant themes emerged:

- Visiting Nursing/Public Health Nursing Practice

During the nineteenth to mid-twentieth centuries, most healthcare in the rural and isolated core of Appalachia was provided in the community instead of in a hospital or doctor's office setting. Up until the early to mid-twentieth century, there were few (if any) professionally educated physicians available. In the absence of physicians, nurses went directly to the patients in the community.

- Outsider/Insider Phenomenon

Many pioneer nurses and doctors who migrated to Appalachia had been born, raised, and educated in large cities outside the region. These nurses and doctors were considered outsiders ("fotched on"—brought in from elsewhere) and viewed with suspicion by local community residents, to the extent that, as outsiders, they had to gain trust and respect in order to be accepted into the community.

- Perseverance, Resilience, and Determination

Nurses practicing in the core of Appalachia frequently had to visit patients by horseback, by mule, or on foot, traveling long distances across mountains and rivers in harsh weather.

- East Coast Connection with a Bellevue Hospital Footprint

Nurses, nurse educators, and nursing superintendents came to Appalachia from hospital training schools in the East and helped establish new hospital training programs for nurses in the core of Appalachia. Bellevue Hospital Training School for Nurses was foundational in

Introduction

its legacy of nursing education for nurses who received their training in the Northeast and were instrumental in creating the basis for professional nurses' training in the core of Appalachia.

- Genesis of Advanced Practice Nursing

Because of the lack of physicians and hospitals in the rural and isolated communities in the Appalachian region, nurses frequently had to perform procedures that were usually outside the practice of nursing and exclusive to medicine. Two examples can be observed in the experiences of Lydia Holman and Mary Breckinridge.

At the turn of the century, Lydia Holman, RN, in Mitchell County, North Carolina, performed procedures that were outside the parameters of nursing practice at the time. She set bones, sutured wounds, pulled teeth, and performed other procedures outside of traditional nursing practice. Later, by the 1920s, due to the absence of locally available physicians, Mary Breckinridge, RN, established the Frontier Nursing Service, providing the valuable aid of professionally trained nurse midwives to deliver babies and care for mothers in the eastern Kentucky mountains.

It wasn't until decades later that the education and role of advanced practice nurses emerged. While nurses such as Holman and Breckinridge were not labeled advanced practice nurses at the time, their talents and experience frequently went far beyond traditional nursing practice, paving the way for the current role of advanced practice nurse.

I

Geographic Setting and Early Healthcare

Geography of Southern Appalachia and Early Settlers

The entire Appalachian region of the United States spans more than 205,000 square miles and encompasses portions of New York, Pennsylvania, Ohio, Maryland, South Carolina, North Carolina, Alabama, Georgia, Mississippi, Kentucky, Tennessee, and Virginia, as well as all of West Virginia. Due to the region's size and diversity, the Appalachian Regional Commission created three subregions: Northern, Southern, and Central Appalachia (Appalachian Regional Commission, n.d.).

This history is geographically centered in the core of Appalachia, a subregion of Southern and Central Appalachia, defined and described by John Williams (Williams, 2002). The states and their Appalachian core counties in this history include the following:

- Georgia (northwestern section of the state) counties: Whitfield, White, Walker, Union, Towns, Rabun, Pickens, Fannin, Floyd, Gilmer, Gordon, Habersham, Murray, Lumpkin, Bartow, Catoosa, Chattooga, Dade, and Dawson.
- Kentucky (eastern section of the state) counties: Magoffin, Martin, Menifee, Morgan, Owsley, Perry, Pike, Powell, Rowan, Whitley, Wolfe, Lee, Bell, Boyd, Breathitt, Carter, Clay, Elliott, Estill, Floyd, Harlan, Laurel, Johnson, Knott, Knox, Jackson, Lawrence, Leslie, Letcher, and McCreary.
- North Carolina (western section of the state) counties: Alleghany, Ashe, Avery, Buncombe, Cherokee, Clay, Graham,

Haywood, Henderson, Macon, Madison, Mitchell, Swain, Transylvania, Watauga, Wilkes, Yancey, McDowell, Jackson, Caldwell, and Burke.
- Tennessee (eastern section of the state) counties: Rhea, Roane, Scott, Sequatchie, Sullivan, Unicoi, Union, Van Buren, Washington, Loudon, Anderson, Bledsoe, Bradley, Campbell, Claiborne, Cumberland, Fentress, Grainger, Grundy, Hamblen, Hamilton, Hancock, Hawkins, Jefferson, Johnson, Knox, McMinn, Marion, Meigs, Morgan, Monroe, Cocke, Sevier, Carter, Greene, Blount, and Polk.
- Virginia (western/southwestern section of the state) counties: Pulaski, Russell, Scott, Smyth, Tazewell, Washington, Wise, Wythe, Alleghany, Carroll, Montgomery, Grayson, Giles, Floyd, Dickenson, Craig, Buchanan, Bland, Bath, Lee, Highland, Washington, Rockbridge, and Botetourt. Roanoke was added to the list since it is located in a border county of the Appalachian core region and served as a central hub for the southwest Virginia (core) region during the late nineteenth and early twentieth centuries.
- West Virginia (majority of the state) counties: Raleigh, Preston, Pocahontas, Nicholas, Monroe, Monongalia, Mingo, Mercer, Marion, McDowell, Logan, Lincoln, Kanawha, Greenbrier, Randolph, Gilmer, Fayette, Clay, Braxton, Boone, Wyoming, Barbour, Taylor, Webster, Wayne/Cabell, Upshur, Tucker, Summers, Lewis, Harrison, Hardy, Pendleton, Mineral, Grant, and Hampshire.

Note: There were several counties in each of the above states that were contiguous to and representative of the core Appalachian counties and have been included in this history (Mapping Appalachia, n.d.).

Early Settlers of Southern Appalachia

The earliest inhabitants of Southern Appalachia were Native Americans (Zeigler & Grosscup, 1883). By the early to mid-eighteenth century, European settlers of Scot, Irish, Scotch-Irish, and German ancestry had made their way into the region and became known as the "Southern Mountaineers" or "Southern Highlanders." These early settlers (sometimes referred to as "mountain dwellers") were described as self-sufficient, living in isolation, and shut off by the mountains (Fox,

I. Geographic Setting and Early Healthcare

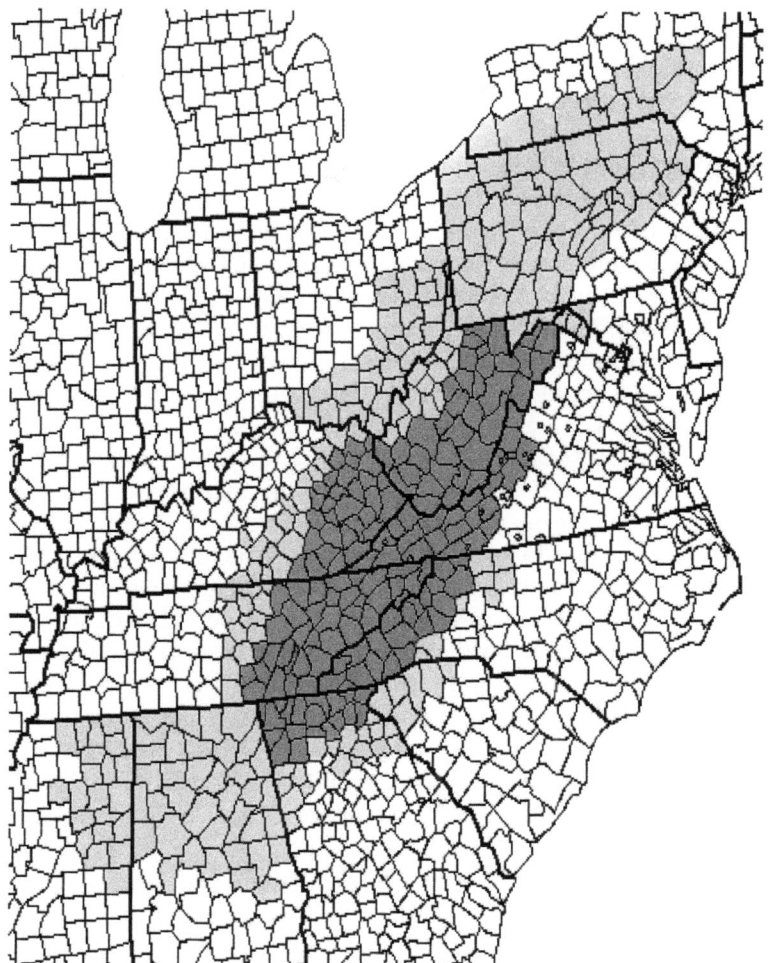

Map of Appalachian core counties (S. Loury/M. Street).

1901; Yarnell, 1998). They were known to be a resilient people who used their skills, crafts, talents, and traditions in agriculture and lumber, making by hand what they needed to sustain themselves, sell, or barter (Roberts, 1988). The settlers brought with them their ancestral beliefs, values, and traditions, which were then passed down from generation to generation. They viewed themselves as having self-worth as long as they could own a small plot of land that was usually bequeathed to their descendants. Considered clannish, the settlers of Southern Appalachia kept to themselves and were skeptical of all outsiders. It took a newcomer time to gain trust and respect before being accepted into the local community (Roberts & Roberts, 1970).

Until the point in time when pioneers pushed westward to discover new land in the nation, Southern Appalachia was considered the westernmost frontier of the United States. The region was described as a land that consisted of mountains, valleys, plateaus, and mineral springs. In addition, Southern Appalachia was viewed as one of the poorest regions of the United States until after the Civil War and the beginning of industrialization with railroads, coal mining, and lumber industries (Campbell, 1921; Dunaway, 1996; Wilson, 1914). During the eighteenth and early nineteenth centuries, Appalachia was similar to other rural regions of the United States where rivers, bridle paths, and Native American trails served as access to and from communities, including trade and transportation. In 1769, Daniel Boone forged a trail across the North Carolina mountains that may possibly have been the first trail in the Southern Appalachia region. In 1778, a wagon road was created (Arthur, 1914). During the first quarter of the nineteenth century, new road construction began, but it was random and disorganized due to the geography of the region, where mountains, cliffs, rocks, streams, and rivers were barriers to construction (Arthur, 1914; Campbell, 1921). At best, the roads were often narrow, steep, and rocky. By the 1820s, turnpikes, created to help bridge the larger and smaller communities across Southern Appalachia, had begun to emerge. Stagecoaches took passengers across the region and frequently brought patients from other parts of the United States to therapeutic mineral springs scattered throughout Southern Appalachia. The arrival of the railroad during the 1850s brought the world closer to Appalachia, though most railroad networks and towns were located in the more urban areas of the region, leaving many small, rural Appalachian communities isolated and difficult to reach. Given the lack of roads or rail in these remote communities, the most feasible methods of travel over the rugged mountainous terrain were usually by horse, by mule, or on foot.

By the 1880s, dirt and gravel roads had been built to facilitate local travel to and from remote rural communities. However, roads frequently became impassable, turning into mud during heavy rains or dust during the hot and often dry summers (Hamilton, 2018). Many of the isolated

I. Geographic Setting and Early Healthcare

rural communities remained inaccessible or difficult to reach well into the mid-twentieth century, leaving residents without access to important resources, including physicians, hospitals, or professional healthcare. As a result, community residents relied on lay or granny doctors, midwives, and family caregiving (Crowe-Carraco, 1978).

Although the 1920s and 1930s brought some improvement with road and rail in the Southern Appalachian region, transportation to and from the very rural and isolated communities remained problematic. Many of these communities were located twenty miles or more from the rail network. In 1921, a visitor to Madison County, North Carolina, described her journey to reach the rural community of White Rock:

> I rode up a narrow trail in the North Carolina Mountains. I was some twenty miles from the nearest railroad. The road had been dwindling steadily for some hours, as it took its way over ridge after ridge, followed stream after stream, crossed bridge after bridge and climbed steadily toward the land of the sky. About us for hours had been only the precipitous landscape of the mountains: rocky creeks and steep hills, soft, weather beaten log cabins set along watercourses that scarred the wooded slopes, a changing vista of forest and sky [Bellamy, 1921, p. 3].

The visitor further described her surroundings as

> poor but beautiful log cabins, with little patches of tobacco and corn, set in remote wooded, mountain valleys, cut off from the outside world by impassable roads and creeks, and inhabited by a pure Scotch-Irish race struggling against primitive conditions, but possessed of some of the best blood of America, if only given a chance [Bellamy, 1921, p. 5].

North Carolina was not the only state in Southern Appalachia with geographic challenges and transportation issues. One Kentucky nurse described similar challenges in trying to reach an elderly couple who needed care in Leslie County, Kentucky. The couple resided on Beech Fork: "You could go six miles on a horse or thirty miles in the jeep. Needless to say, I took the horse" (Montell, 2015).

Traditional Healers, Early Physicians and Medical Training

During the eighteenth and nineteenth centuries, residents in the rural and remote communities in the core of Appalachia relied on the only resources they had for healthcare. As early as 1770, there were providers whom local community residents of Southern Appalachia called "doctors"; however, these individuals were not professionally trained. Prior to the nineteenth century, like other rural regions of the United States, most areas of Southern Appalachia lacked access to professionally trained physicians, which left the care of its residents to family members, lay healers, self-taught/professed doctors, "mountain grannies" or granny midwives and trusted members of the community (Barney, 1996; Campbell, 1921).

Although formal medical training in the United States can be traced back to 1765, most medical schools were located in large eastern cities. During the early part of the nineteenth century, formal medical education had begun to expand across the United States; however, the premier medical training institutions were still found in cities such as New York, Philadelphia, Boston, and Baltimore. At this time, medical schools began to emerge in the South, including Nashville and Memphis, Tennessee. In the mid-nineteenth century, medical care provided by doctors in the rural isolated areas of the nation, including the Appalachian region, was still described as "primitive." Many of the local doctors in the Southern Appalachian region lacked formal medical education and had to rely on limited knowledge, minimal equipment, and what medicines they had (Barney, 2000). Any type of formal medical education in the rural areas was either nonexistent or minimal at best. Further, the medical schools that did exist in Southern Appalachia were located in the large urban areas of the region, which made it difficult for those who lived in the rural and isolated Southern Appalachian communities to further their education.

Many of those in the rural communities who aspired to become doctors did not have the financial resources to travel to and attend medical school in a large city. As a result, they were excluded from the benefit of formal professional medical education and were generally self-trained (Barney, 2000). If they were trained at all, the training was considered rudimentary, consisting of a few medical courses or using Gunn's 1830 *Domestic Medicine* book as a basis for their medical knowledge. In many cases, these primitive or "self-professed" doctors may have received their medical knowledge working as apprentices under another self-professed physician; however, once "trained," they were practicing without formal medical education, a degree, or license (Barney, 2000). The early self-trained doctors were also referred to as "folk" doctors, using traditional remedies and Native American medicines as treatments. These individuals were nevertheless trusted in

I. Geographic Setting and Early Healthcare

their communities because they were residents, and the procedures they performed (which usually included herbal and folk medicine remedies) were embraced. For decades, Appalachian residents had relied on self-professed doctors and healers, granny midwives, "mountain doctors," home remedies, and herbal medicines and tonics because they had not yet been exposed to formal scientific medicine by professionally trained physicians (Barney, 1996).

In the absence of a professionally educated doctor to care for illness, injuries, or other medical issues in the community, most residents of rural Southern Appalachia frequently turned to family members for remedies that had been handed down by their ancestors, local folk healers, "mountain doctors," and granny midwives. This practice continued well into the twentieth century, and some of those early remedies and cures are still used or practiced today. Some residents have resumed the practice of herbal folk medicine (or herbal "doctoring") because of what they learned as children (Deskins, 1990). Folk healers continued to practice healing using herbal medicines that were handed down by their ancestors, who had first learned these techniques from local Native Americans (Green, 1978). The practice of folk healing remained prevalent in the Appalachian region throughout the nineteenth century. Some folk healers were thought to have supernatural powers, while other healers could be identified by their treatment for specific conditions or ailments—for example, thrush, warts, and burns (Cavender, 2003). The yarb (or herb) doctors used plants as remedies to treat or cure illness and would often combine plants and herbs with supernatural techniques or magic. Some granny midwives would use medicinal plants for healing and frequently served as yarb doctors as well. These healers were all untrained and mostly self-professed doctors (Cavender, 2003; Jones, 1949).

Along with folk healers and self-professed doctors, granny midwives were considered a prominent source of healthcare in the community. Granny midwives were women who attended and conducted the delivery of babies in the community. In addition to delivering babies, the granny midwife frequently treated other members of the family. Although not professionally trained, granny midwives (sometimes called "granny doctors") were the only source of medical care available to residents in the rural and isolated areas of the Southern Appalachian region. To comfort or heal their patients, the granny midwives commonly relied on herbal and traditional remedies, folk beliefs, and spirituality for healing (Green, 1978).

Early Physicians and Medical Training in the Core of Appalachia

Formal medical training in the United States can be traced back to the eighteenth century and took place in the larger cities of the United States, including New York, Philadelphia, Boston, and Baltimore. Some individuals in the Southern Appalachia region were fortunate to have the necessary financial resources and support to attend a premier training school in a large city. Dr. Joseph Orrin Wilcox (born in 1844 in Ashe County, North Carolina) aspired to be a doctor and was one of the few individuals from the region with resources that enabled him to attend Johns Hopkins Medical School in Baltimore, Maryland; he graduated sometime before 1870. Dedicated to bringing much-needed healthcare back to his home, he returned to rural Ashe County and established a medical practice in his own community. Not only was Wilcox the sole physician in the North Fork area of the New River in North Carolina, but he also became known as an excellent practitioner and built a large practice in northwest North Carolina and eastern Tennessee. Keenly aware of the limitations experienced by those in the region who aspired to become doctors but lacked the resources to attend medical school, Wilcox decided to open a medical school on his own home property near Creston in Ashe County. Based on what he had learned in his own medical education and training at Johns Hopkins, Wilcox provided medical lectures to the students and assigned them to the patients he visited, at which time, under his personal guidance and supervision, they would make diagnoses and provide treatment. His medical school was short lived, but it served to illustrate the resourcefulness of a local physician in his attempt to provide professional medical care for the region (Fletcher, 1963; History of the Worth Family, n.d.; Pittard, 2016).

While Wilcox had established his medical practice in the same community in which he lived, the issue remained that wider access to medical care and education during this early period was considerably limited in the core of Appalachia. Unlike Wilcox, who was a local member of the community where he had established his practice, most physicians who eventually came to practice medicine in the core of Appalachia were from regions beyond Southern Appalachia and had been formally educated in large eastern cities. Considered "outsiders," many of these physicians were hesitant to permanently settle in the rural Southern Appalachian region because of economic reasons (patients

I. Geographic Setting and Early Healthcare

often had trouble paying for medical care), rural isolation, and the community residents' preference for local trusted healers and innate distrust of outsiders (Barney, 1996). The physicians who did relocate to Southern Appalachia were referred to by local residents as "furriners" (foreigners) or "fotched-on" (outsiders), meaning brought in or "fetched" from outside the region (Bellamy, 1921). These "outsider" physicians were frequently viewed with suspicion by the local community residents. The "fotched-on" doctor had to earn the trust and respect of the community residents before he or she would be accepted into the community.

Laurel, a small remote community in Madison County, North Carolina, was a prime example of community distrust when, in 1914, Dr. George Packard, a "fotched-on" doctor from Boston, was sent to Laurel by the Presbyterian Church Board of Home Missions in New York. The only connection to the Laurel community of this "fotched-on" doctor was through Frances Goodrich, a Presbyterian missionary; otherwise, he was basically unknown to the community residents. Because Packard was an outsider, the community residents viewed him with distrust, which included Granny Banks, the local "mountain doctor." Granny Banks was never formally educated as a physician but had been taking care of the Laurel community for many years and considered herself an old-time mountain doctor. Her methods of healing included roots, herbs, and prayers. When Packard arrived, Banks resented the intrusion of this new "fotched-on" medical doctor with his "fancy" education. Banks believed that her seventy-eight years of experience and general aptitude outweighed four years of medical education. According to local legend, every time Granny Banks and the doctor passed one another on the road, Banks greeted him with "Go to Hell" (Tweed, 2016).

In the beginning, the community residents were also suspicious of Packard—that is, until a medical emergency arose when a local community leader developed appendicitis and immediate surgery was required. Due to the urgent nature of the leader's condition and the inability to move the patient to a hospital several miles away, Packard had to perform an emergency appendectomy in the leader's own cabin. The patient was placed on the kitchen table, the only possible surface available for surgery. A lamp from the church was used to provide light, and the church minister administered the ether. Looking through the cabin door and windows, local residents observed the procedure. The surgery was a success, and Packard remained to ensure the patient was out of danger. The community leader had survived, and Packard gained the

Appalachian Nursing

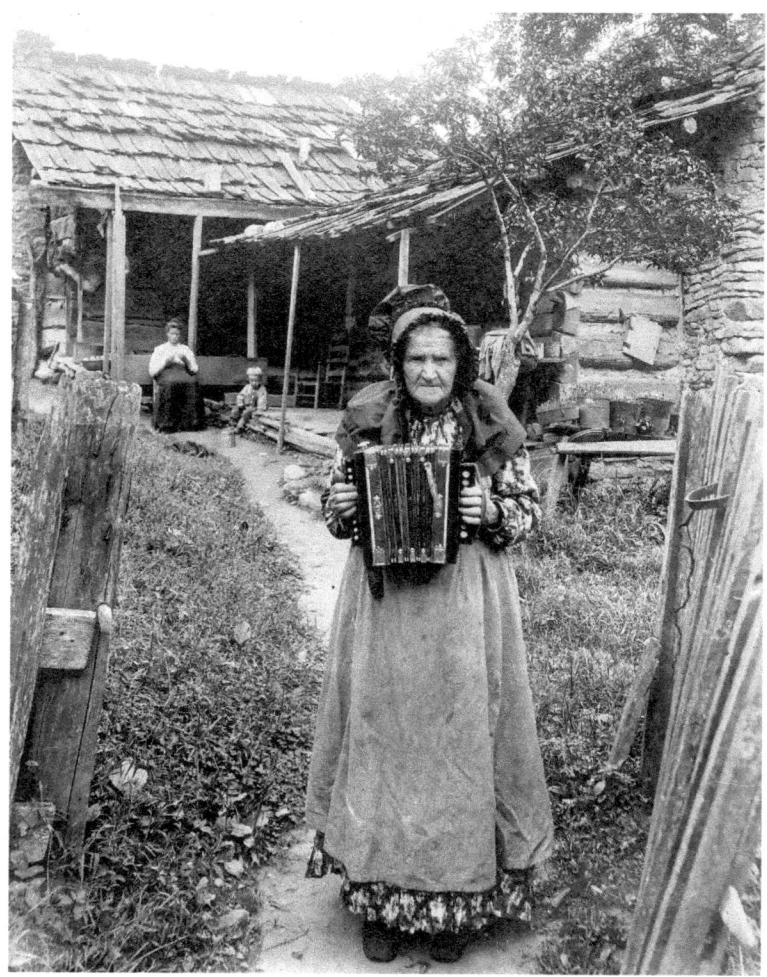

Ealy (Granny) Banks, "mountain doctor" (in foreground), Laurel, North Carolina, c. 1840 (courtesy Southern Highland Craft Guild, Archives Library, Asheville, North Carolina).

confidence and respect of the Laurel community. From that moment forward, Packard was accepted into the community and became a revered and well-respected community member as well as their trusted doctor, even providing medical care for Granny Banks when her own health deteriorated (Bellamy, 1921; Tweed, 2016).

I. Geographic Setting and Early Healthcare

Early Remedies and Healing Practices

Remedies

Although isolated from more populated areas, residents of Southern Appalachia experienced the same illnesses, injuries, and medical conditions as did the rest of the U.S. population. Remedies they used to treat common ailments were usually based on tradition and the natural or supernatural beliefs of their early settler ancestors that had been passed down from one generation to the next. These remedies sometimes merged with the influence of the region's Native American remedies and their use of local indigenous plants that included goldenseal, sassafras, bloodroot, horsemint, boneset, and others.

While not an exhaustive list, common herbal remedies in the region included the following:

- Cally root was used to promote sleep, treat colds, and colic.
- Bruised peach tree, plantain, or sweet potato leaves, dipped in boiling water and cooled, were applied to the skin to soothe aching heels.
- Pennyrile (pennyroyal), rosemary, or ginger tea was used to treat stomachaches; if that did not work, chewing sweet calamus root was tried to expel the gas. Pennyroyal tea was also useful for breaking fevers or treating painful menstrual cramps.
- Goldenseal was used for mouth and throat sores and many other ailments.
- Boneset tea had numerous purposes, including being used as a diaphoretic to "sweat out" chest colds as well as an agent to induce vomiting.
- Clover blossom (red blooms) tea was used for curing "all diseases."
- White clover blossom tea served as a blood purifier.
- Sassafras tea had many uses, including blood purifier, general spring tonic, and (in a weak solution) eye wash. Sassafras could also be made into a poultice for a stye by scraping and scalding freshly dug roots. Sometimes babies were given a spoonful of sassafras tea for colic.
- Castor oil was often used for fever blisters along with mild food and senna tea several times a day, followed by chewing senna leaves each day until healed.

- Upset stomachs were treated by chewing the bark of a slippery elm or any other tree as long as it was peeled from the south side of a tree that grew on a hill's north side (Cavender, 2003). Many of these remedies are still used today.

Healing Practices

Childbirth in Southern Appalachia, considered a blessing, usually began at a very early age. It was not uncommon for girls to be married by the age of 14; many women went on to give birth to ten or more children. For childbirth pain and healing, herbal and folk remedies were the usual treatment of choice. One practice for addressing labor pains involved placing an axe (or sharp object) under the bed. It was thought to not only relieve the pain but also stop hemorrhaging (Montell, 2015).

To hasten labor, sometimes a quill filled with red pepper or gunpowder was placed in the pregnant woman's nose so that she would sneeze. In cases of mastitis, cow manure was spread on the mother's breasts ("Old Time Appalachian," 2017).

Numerous remedies were provided for colic. One remedy was to pass the child from mother to father three times around a table leg, under a horse, or around a split seedling. Sometimes the child was given catnip tea or a teaspoon of whiskey "scorched" (cooked) to burn off the alcohol (Cavender, 2003). To remove a membrane that formed over the larynx as a result of croup, midwife Cora Reeves of North Carolina recommend giving the child a "little" lamp oil every few minutes to "cut" and eliminate the membrane (Cavender, 2005; Cora Ennis Smith Reeves, n.d.).

One common belief regarding thrush (thrash) was that it could be cured by a "seventh son"—that is, the seventh son in a line (without any female siblings) born to a "seventh son," believed to have an inherent special power to cure thrush in babies. The child would be taken to the "seventh son," who would then blow into the baby's mouth, after which the baby would be cured (Cavender, 2003; Whaley, personal communication, April 20, 2018).

Other common medical practices for both adults and children included using vinegar-infused brown paper as a remedy for sprains and poultices for infections. Sliding a knife, scissors, or other flat metal down a patient's back was done to stop a nosebleed. Remedies for fever, pneumonia, muscle aches, and headaches were based on "burning" the problem out of the body. This could include the topical application of mustard seed, cayenne pepper, Spanish fly, or other substance that would irritate the skin (Cavender, 2003).

Asafetida, which came from the rhizome of ferula or roots from similar plants, had a strong, unpleasant odor. It was placed in a small bag and worn around the neck to ward off illness. The cally plant was frequently used to treat colds and colic. Sumac (white shumake) was used to treat burns; Indian hemp root was infused in whiskey to treat "sun pain"—that is, migraine headache (Bolyard, 1981).

Madstones (or bezoars) were considered a remedy to treat infections. They were round, stone-like objects consisting of calcium and animal hair that were found in the stomachs or intestines of deer and bears. Madstones were placed on wounds to draw out the poison or infection (Cavender, 2003; Whaley, personal communication, April 20, 2018).

Patent Medicines

Patent medicines became a popular remedy across the nation (including Southern Appalachia) throughout the eighteenth through mid-twentieth centuries. Sold in bottles and marketed under proprietary names, these elixirs and tonics contained a mixture of compounds with an unusually high concentration of alcohol, and frequently opium or cocaine (Hagley Museum and Library, n.d.). There were a number of patent medicine companies established in Southern Appalachia during the nineteenth century. The most well known were:

- The Chattanooga Medicine Company, established in 1870, famous for its Wine of Cardui and Black Draught
- East Tennessee Medicine Company of Jonesborough, Tennessee, established in 1890 and known for indigestion relief and cough syrup
- Landrum and Litchfield of Abingdon, Virginia, established in 1870 and known for its compound of minerals in a tonic form as a restorative tonic
- Andrews Manufacturing Company, founded by Ernest Andrews in 1892, who created a number of mixtures; among the best known was Andrews Winde of Life Root (National Museum of American History, n.d.)

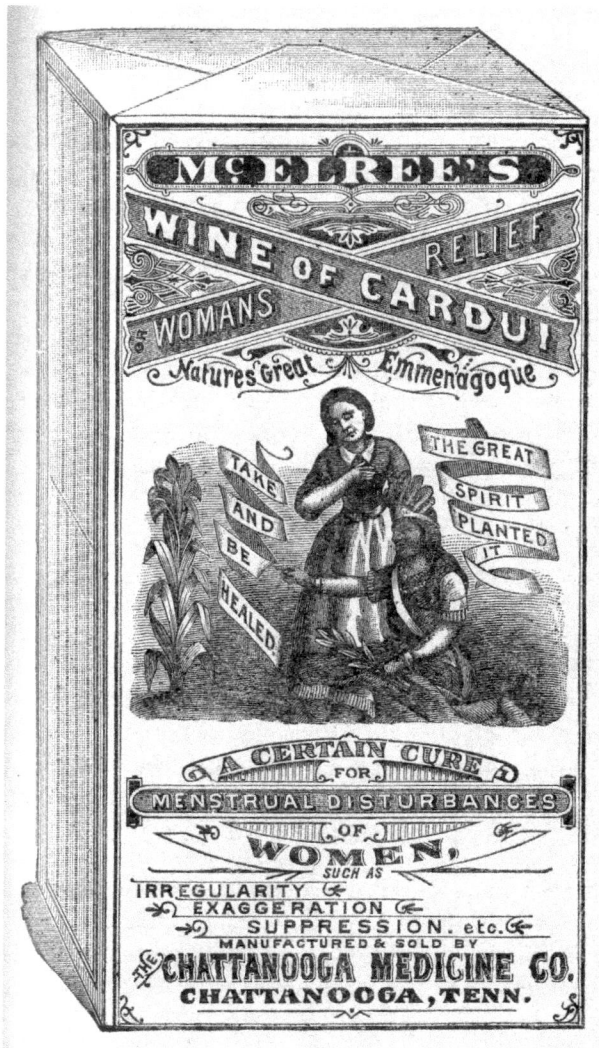

McElree's Wine of Cardui ad, c. 1894 (R.L. McElree Chattanooga Medicine Co., *Home Treatment of Female Diseases* [booklet]).

These medicines were usually sold through medicine shows, from the backs of wagons, and through advertising. Most were promoted as a cure for specific ailments, such as dyspepsia, catarrh, women's

I. Geographic Setting and Early Healthcare

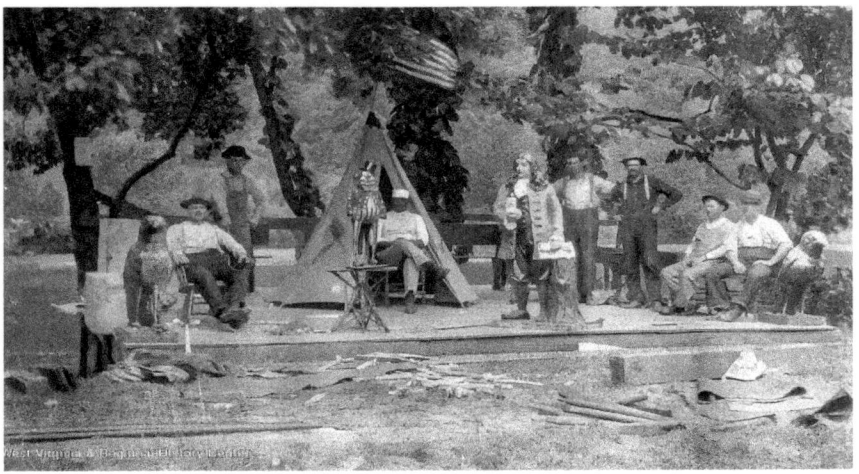

Medicine show stage near Morgantown, West Virginia, n.d. (West Virginia and Regional History Center, West Virginia University Libraries).

complaints, or general malaise (or sometimes a combination of more than one ailment). Chattanooga Medicine Company was a large manufacturer of patent medicines. From the late nineteenth through mid-twentieth centuries, McElree's Wine of Cardui, one of the company's earlier medicines, was marketed as a tonic for women's ailments. It was extensively advertised in numerous magazines and periodicals during that period. Wine of Cardui contained 19 percent ethyl alcohol (National Museum of American History, n.d.).

Medicine shows, designed to sell patent medicines to the public, were very popular during the nineteenth century. They created a carnival-like atmosphere in towns across the United States, and in the rural and isolated regions of Southern Appalachia, they sometimes provided a community's only entertainment. The proprietary medicine company hired showmen and musicians to entertain the crowd, along with a "pitchman" to promote and sell the product. Most of the medicines were promoted as tonics or elixirs, intended to make individuals feel better, and as a cure for almost any ailment. Usually advertised as medical remedies, these concoctions consisted of vegetable compounds and alcohol as high as 19–20 percent (listed as a preservative). In addition, many of these mixtures contained opium, cocaine, or morphine (International Independent Showmen's Museum, n.d.).

Appalachian Nursing

In addition to medicine shows, advertisements for a variety of medicines, concoctions, and cures could be found in popular magazines. Written endorsements were frequently used as advertising to promote a particular patent medicine. Dr. Pierce's "Favorite Prescription" for women's ailments was a very popular tonic containing lady's slipper root, blue cohosh root, unicorn root, black cohosh root, Oregon grape root, and viburnum (no alcohol). In an 1898 advertisement endorsing Dr. Pierce's "Favorite Prescription," a young mother wrote, "I am now thirty-six years old and have given birth to ten children." She went on to state that after the birth of her twin boys in 1896,

> I was confined to my bed all spring and summer with female complaint; had it so badly I could hardly walk around the house without feeling worse. I did not call my doctors as I had tried the doctors twice before when I was down with the same trouble. ... I had almost lost all hope of being able to do anything.... No one can know the distress of my mind as well as body. Dr. Pierce's Favorite Prescription was the only medicine that seemed to do me any good.... I believe I took eight bottles and then I felt like a different person. I gave birth to another baby and my old complaint came back. I began using the Favorite Prescription and was soon relieved and was able to do my work [*Nebraska State Journal*, 1898, p. 12].

Other medicines, including McElree's Wine of Cardui and Thedford's Black Draught (Chattanooga Medicine Company), were also favorites, as described by M. F., Farabee, Indiana: "I am thirty-seven years of age and have suffered ever since I became a woman until I commenced taking Wine of Cardui. I have used seven bottles and believe I am entirely cured" (McElree, 1894). From Miss A. G., Barren Fork, Arkansas:

> If there was ever a moment in my life before I was eighteen years old that my head did not ache I cannot remember it. I had palpitations of the heart, terrible aches all over, dizziness, fainting spells, back ached constantly, and I felt just almost gone, But thank God! I was saved by some one sending me a package of Black-Draught. Your medicine is truly a great blessing to suffering humanity. I can't recommend it highly enough [McElree, 1894].

Healing Springs

Another form of early healing in the core of Appalachia was found in mineral waters known as "healing springs." During the nineteenth and twentieth centuries, these springs drew many visitors to the region from all over the country. The springs were scattered throughout

I. Geographic Setting and Early Healthcare

Appalachia, differentiated according to the location and minerals found in the local spring waters. Therefore, cures for specific conditions varied. Originally discovered by the Native Americans in the 1700s, some of the most popular springs were located in the western region of Virginia.

One popular spring site, owned by Dr. Goode, was located in Hot Springs, Bath County, Virginia. The water contained sulphate, carbonate of lime, sulphate of soda and magnesia, muriate of iron, carbonic acid gas, nitrogen gas, and sulphuretted hydrogen gas. The temperature of the springs' waters ranged from 98 to 106 degrees (Burke, 1846; McAllister, 2017; Moorman, 1817). A hotel was built, as the springs attracted visitors from other parts of the United States. The visitors traveled by stagecoach to reach the hotel and its springs. There were bathing houses for both male and female visitors and six baths that were supplied by separate springs. Goode collected testimonials from his visitors (Goode, 1839). In an 1833 letter, H. Calloway described the benefit of hot springs:

> In the months of January, 1806, during my attendance on the Virginia Legislature, of which I was then a member, I was very sorely afflicted with an attack of inflammatory rheumatism; and about the first of July, in the same year, after the disease had assumed a chronic state, I arrived at the Hot Springs in Virginia much debilitated requiring two persons to put me in and take me out of the carriage. I remained at the Springs sixty-three days, using the bath once every day except three ... and remained free from that complaint for upwards of twenty years [Goode, 1839, p. 7].

II

The Evolution of Nursing Education and Professional Nursing

The Beginning of Formal Nurses' Training in the United States

In 1860, Florence Nightingale established a program of professional training for nurses at St. Thomas Hospital in London, England. Within the principles of the Nightingale model, the nurse's character was modeled through training in which adherence to order, loyalty, deference to the physician, and constant drilling in proper conduct was emphasized. Nightingale believed that a good training school for nurses should have a suitable administration with medical officers and a superintendent to whom nurses would report. In addition to demonstrating proper conduct, Nightingale felt a nurse must be able to recognize the symptoms and cause of disease. She also emphasized that nursing was an art, and nurses should nurse the individual rather than the illness (Nightingale, 1859).

With the exception of a physician-owned and -operated one-year training program for nurses at the New England Hospital for Women and Children in Boston, Massachusetts, and a sixth-month nurses' training program at Philadelphia Hospital, professional training schools for nurses in the United States did not exist until the first formal training program based on the Nightingale model of professional nursing was established in 1873 at Bellevue Hospital in New York City. Bellevue Hospital was known for treating the poor and immigrant population; however, like many other hospitals during that time, it also had a history of sanitation problems in which conditions of the patients and beds were "unspeakable" (Nightingale, Woolsey, & Hobson, 1950; Stewart,

II. Evolution of Nursing Education/Professional Nursing

1984). When it was decided that a Nightingale-based training school for nurses would be established at Bellevue Hospital, the need and focus on nurse education and training was directed toward improving hospital conditions and outcomes, specified in an early Bellevue Report as two-fold: to "make this great hospital ... a place where the respectable poor could be tenderly and skillfully nursed ... where even the most degraded of paupers would be sure of kindly and patient care" and to train "a band of experienced, obedient, devoted nurses for service in private cases or among the poor" (Stewart, 1984, p. 91).

Formal aims of the Bellevue Training School for Nurses program were:

    1. "To train intelligent women to become skilled hospital nurses ... whose standard of nurses duties would be rigid, thus improving hospital training, not only at Bellevue, but throughout the country.

    2. To train nurses for the proper care of the sick in private families.

    3. To send nurses to the sick poor in their own homes" (Bellevue School of Nursing, 1989, p. 25)

Following the establishment of the Bellevue Training School for Nurses in 1873, two other Nightingale-based nurses' training schools were formed several months later in that same year: the Connecticut Training School for Nurses in New Haven, Connecticut, and the Boston Training School for Nurses at Massachusetts General Hospital in Boston, Massachusetts. The Bellevue, Connecticut, and Boston nursing schools became the original hallmark for Nightingale-based professional nurse training in the United States. Soon after the establishment of those first three institutions in the East, professional training schools for nurses began to open across the United States.

While this development may have been the beginning of professional education for nurses in the United States, it became apparent that room for improvement existed in the formal training of nurses. In spite of Nightingale's influence, nurses' training schools throughout the United States (including the Bellevue, Connecticut, and Boston programs) lacked clear educational standards and rigor in the curricula. In addition, the administrators of hospitals with nurses' training schools had derived a significant benefit by using nursing students as a form of free labor. In 1901, Dr. J. William White, professor of clinical surgery at the University of Pennsylvania, wrote:

Appalachian Nursing

> I know of no exception to the statement that in every instance the addition of a training school to a hospital has increased its efficiency, and in the long run has reduced both its expenses and, what is vastly more important, its mortality. Evidence recently collected shows beyond all question that the material prosperity of the hospital is largely due to the work of the training school ... a definite impetus and advance in hospital work dates from the foundation of trained nursing [White, 1895, p. 3].

Students in other hospital training schools followed an education program similar to those of Bellevue, Connecticut, and Boston (Massachusetts General). Although hospitals may have benefited, this usage of student nurses' labor caused the education of nursing students to become secondary to the operation of the hospital, which was a significant source of concern for nursing leaders. Students in nurses' training programs lived at the hospital and, during the day, spent their time working in the hospital wards while also learning routine nursing skills and how to care for patients. These skills were normally taught by the nurse superintendent of the hospital. In the evenings, students attended medical classes with lectures in physiology, anatomy, and hygiene taught by the hospital physicians. The training school curriculum included observation of the sick, administration of medicines, heat and

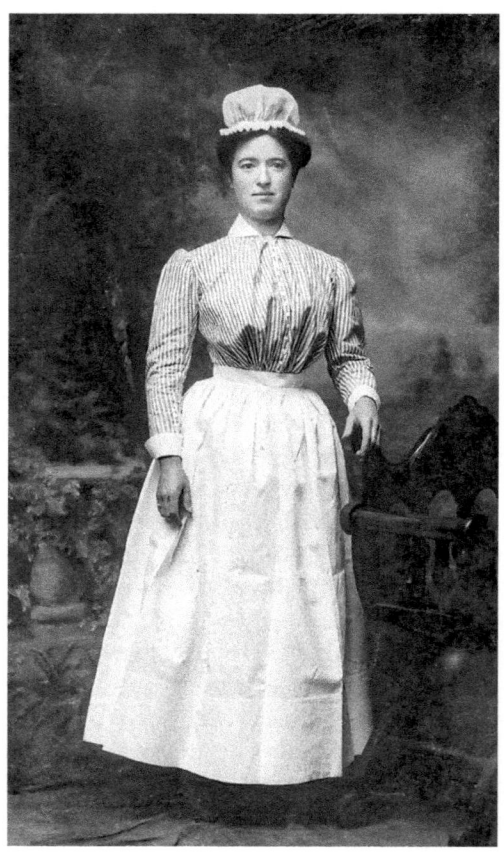

Grace McBride in Bellevue Hospital student uniform, c. 1910 (courtesy Kimberly Kelley, family collection).

II. Evolution of Nursing Education/Professional Nursing

poultice applications, dressing and bandaging of wounds, operations and medical cases, emergencies, monthly (obstetrics) nursing, nursing care of sick children, hygiene, cookery for the sick (dietetics), and hospital management. A significant amount of the students' time, however, was spent tending to the wards of the hospital. This work included housekeeping chores, with a substantial focus on cleanliness of the patient room and the hospital ward itself. Students scuttled coal, swept the floors, cleaned the rooms, and performed other domestic duties (Bellevue Training School for Nurses, 1878; Snively, 1894).

Along with tending to the wards at Bellevue Hospital, a curricular subject of special importance in Bellevue's Training School for Nurses

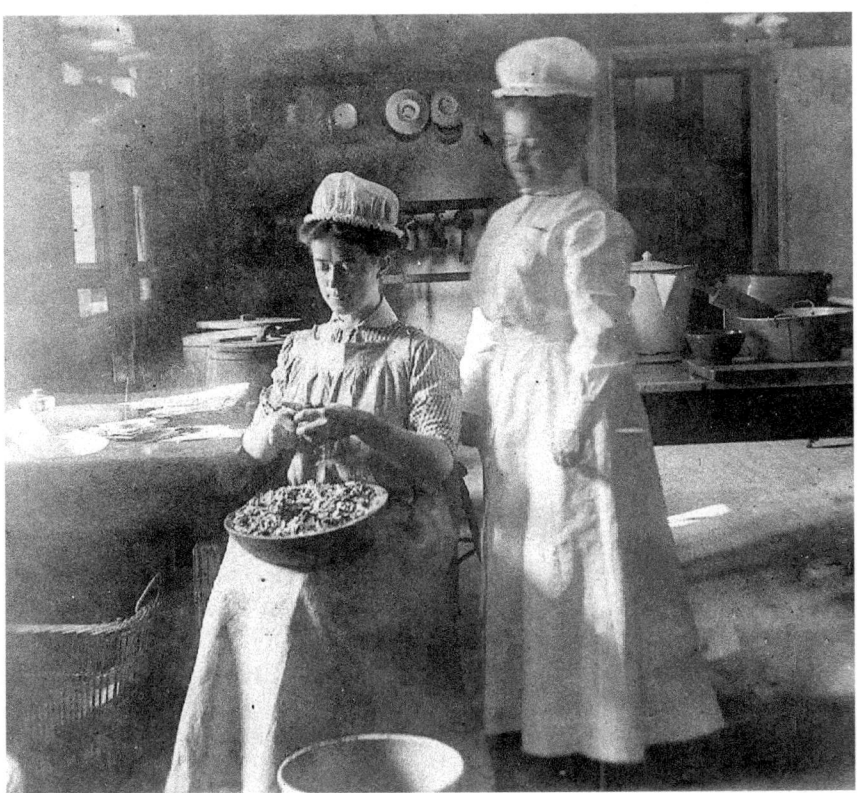

Grace McBride (seated) in Bellevue Hospital kitchen with nursing instructor, c. 1910 (courtesy Kimberly Kelley, family collection).

was the course in "dietetics," in which nursing students were taught how to prepare a variety of foods specific to the dietary needs of the patients. The emphasis on dietetics as part of the nurses' training program was illustrated in a 1910 letter from Grace McBride, superintendent of nurses at Highlands Sanitarium in Chattanooga, Tennessee. As a student in Bellevue's Training School for Nurses, McBride had written a letter to her mother describing her dietetics class:

> Today I went on duty in the diet kitchen and my work was to make the custards and other desserts. I made forty bowls of custard, about twenty of junket and about twenty five of lemon jelly or gelatine. Was off duty from 12 to 1:30 in the afternoon. In the afternoon I picked chicken off the bones for the creamed chicken we make tomorrow and put away the pans and kettles we used this afternoon. Then was off duty at five o'clock. That was not such hard work, much easier than we get on the wards.... Just wish you could watch us in the diet kitchen. I use about a hundred eggs to make the custards and they look nice when they are all done and put out on the long table [McBride, 1910, p. 10].

Early Nursing Education in the Core of Appalachia

Although there was a growing number of nurses' training schools across the United States, prior to the twentieth century, access to such schools in the core of Appalachia remained limited, especially for those who resided in the rural and isolated sections of Southern Appalachian. Young women in the core of Appalachia who wanted to become nurses frequently had to travel long distances for their training. Similar to the issue of limited access to early medical education, nurses' training programs had been established in hospitals located in the larger, more populated or major cities of the United States (New York, Baltimore, Boston, Philadelphia, etc.). This arrangement left rural communities in the core of Appalachia with limited access to not only hospitals but also nursing education, which posed a challenge for individuals in the region who wanted to become nurses but did not have the necessary resources or ability to travel outside the core of Appalachia. It wasn't until the very late 1890s to early 1900s that nurses' training programs began to appear in the Appalachian core region. Prior to 1900, the earliest known

II. Evolution of Nursing Education/Professional Nursing

formal nurses' training schools in existence in the core of Appalachia were located in the following places:

Kentucky
- Berea (Appalachian core border) established 1898: Berea College Training School for Nurses

North Carolina
- Asheville, established 1896: Memorial Mission Hospital School of Nursing

Tennessee
- Chattanooga, established 1899: Baroness Erlanger Training School for Nurses

Virginia
- Roanoke (border county), established 1899: Roanoke Hospital Training School for Nurses

West Virginia
- Charleston, established 1898: Charleston General Hospital Training School for Nurses

Each of these nurses' training schools also went on to achieve formal NLNE accreditation in 1938 (National League of Nursing Education, 1939).

During the late nineteenth and early twentieth centuries, seeking to improve access to healthcare for residents in the more rural and isolated communities in the core of Appalachia, physicians would frequently establish small hospitals and clinics. As a way to staff their hospitals, these physicians created their own nurses' training programs. These training programs helped supply their hospitals with nursing students, who became a convenient and free form of labor. The main problem with the doctor-run training schools was that the programs were physician based and lacked standards, consistency, and appropriate curricula, which nurse leaders in the region found problematic. The programs were frequently disorganized (with little to no attention to Nightingale principles), consisted of few education classes and long hours of work, and were usually short lived.

There was, however, one doctor-owned hospital with a nurses' training program in a small town in northwest Georgia that proved to be something of an exception. Until 1908, there were no known hospital nurses' training schools in Georgia's Appalachian core region.

The majority of hospitals and nurses' training schools in Georgia were located in the larger cities (Atlanta, Augusta, Macon, and Savannah), miles away from the Appalachian core counties in northwest Georgia. Because of the need for medical care in that region, Harbin Hospital was established in 1908 by the Harbin brothers (Drs. R.M. and W.P. Harbin), both of whom had graduated in 1897 from Bellevue Hospital Medical College in New York City. Not only did their new hospital provide needed healthcare for the community in Rome (Floyd County), Georgia, but the doctors also added a nurses' training program, and, in 1909, the Harbin Hospital Training School for Nurses was established. This institution was considered the only professional nurses' training school in the Georgia core region of Appalachia during the early twentieth century. In addition, it was accredited by the Georgia State Board of Nurse Examiners in 1922 (American Nurses Association, 1922).

Nursing Organizations, Reports, and Registration

During the late nineteenth and early twentieth centuries, nursing organizations had begun to develop in the United States. Two key organizations that had a significant impact on nursing education and nursing practice emerged, known today as the National League for Nursing (NLN) and American Nurses Association (ANA).

The years 1873–1900 saw the genesis of training programs for nurses throughout the United States. Prior to 1873, the concept of a professionally trained nurse whose education was based on Nightingale principles was unheard of in the United States. Anyone could call themselves a nurse. The year 1873 had marked the beginning of professional nurses' training in the United States when the first three training schools based on Nightingale principles were established at hospitals in New York, Connecticut, and Massachusetts. Within a short period of time, more professional nurses' training schools began to emerge across the United States. As noted previously, these early training schools for nurses provided hospitals with student nurse labor and were favorably viewed as a financial benefit to the hospitals because of the services the students could provide throughout their training program. While considered a useful resource for the hospital, the actual education of nurses became secondary to the hospital's service needs. Although based on

II. Evolution of Nursing Education/Professional Nursing

Nightingale principles, most of the nurses' training programs throughout the United States lacked educational and legal standards and consistency. Many of the training programs were haphazardly implemented, with a primary focus on the needs of the hospital rather than those of the students. Hospital administrators and physicians directed the student training and their duties in the hospital.

By 1889, nurse leaders across the United States had begun to discuss their concerns about the lack of standardization in nursing education, the use of student nurses to provide excessive free service to hospitals, legal safeguards in nursing practice, and the need to protect students as well as patients. Concerned about the lack of consistent instruction in nurses' training schools across the United States, these nurse leaders felt strongly that there needed to be standards in professional nurse education, appropriate curricula, and suitable clinical training of all nurses. These leaders also believed legislation to protect the public from poorly prepared nurses was vital. They agreed there should be a system of examination with registration so that, in order to practice, nurse graduates would be required to meet specific standards set by the profession (Flanagan, 1976). In addition to expressing concerns about curriculum standardization and professionalism in nursing programs, these same leaders continued to vocalize their concern that students in the hospital setting had become a cheap and convenient labor force. The service needs of the hospital overrode educational requirements, and there were no clear standards regarding the amount of work expected of a student. In addition to taking care of patients, students were required to maintain the environment of the hospital and provide housekeeping, food preparation, and laundry services. They worked long hours, balancing a seven-day work week with evening lectures to attend after working all day.

The 1893 World's Fair in Chicago provided the setting and opportunity for a national discussion among nurse leaders that ultimately resulted in two organized movements to address the concerns about nursing education and professional practice. Key issues were identified and brought forward by nurse leaders during the initial meeting. Although education and professionalism in nursing practice overlapped to a certain extent, they also occurred in concert with one another. One movement had a concentrated focus on the improvement and standardization of nursing education, from which the National League for Nursing (NLN) emerged. The other movement focused on professional practice and demonstration of competence through registration of nurses before they could begin practicing in the profession. That movement resulted in the American Nurses Association (ANA).

National League for Nursing

The National League for Nursing (NLN) began as the American Society of Superintendents of Training Schools for Nurses. During the 1893 World's Fair, 15 superintendents of nurses' training schools met at St. Luke's Hospital in Chicago, Illinois. Voicing concerns about the disorganized education and practice of nurses, the superintendents formed the first formal nursing organization in the United States: the American Society of Superintendents of Training Schools for Nurses. The superintendents of nurses' training schools present at the initial 1893 meeting included the following women:

- Anna Alston, Mount Sinai Training School, New York
- Lucy Bannister, Wisconsin Training School, Milwaukee
- Ella Betts, Homoeopathic Hospital, Brooklyn, New York
- Louise Darche, New York City Training School, Blackwell's Island
- Mary Davis, University Hospital, Philadelphia, Pennsylvania
- Lavinia Dock, formerly of Johns Hopkins Hospital, Baltimore, Maryland
- Mary Greenwood, Jewish Hospital, Cincinnati, Ohio
- Isabel Hampton, Johns Hopkins Hospital, Baltimore, Maryland
- Katherine Lett, St. Luke's Hospital, Chicago, Illinois
- Mary McKechnie, City Hospital, Louisville, Kentucky
- A.E. Nourse, Michael Reese Hospital, Chicago, Illinois
- Sophia Palmer, Garfield Memorial Hospital, Washington, D.C.
- C.E.M. Somerville, General Hospital, Lawrence, Massachusetts
- Irene Sutliffe, New York Hospital, New York
- Elsie Wallace, Children's Hospital, San Francisco, California

The main goals of the American Society of Superintendents of Training Schools for Nurses were focused on:

1. Higher minimum entrance requirements for entry into a nurse training program
2. Improvement of living and working conditions for students in nurses' training programs

II. Evolution of Nursing Education/Professional Nursing

3. Increased opportunities for postgraduate nurses with additional specialized training courses and programs (National League of Nursing, 2018, p. 11)

Isabel Hampton chaired the development of the organization and the outlining of its purpose. Anna Alston of the Mount Sinai Training School was elected president in 1893, and in 1894 she led the first convention of the Superintendents of Training Schools for Nurses that was held in New York City, where the organization's bylaws and constitution, and development of its overall objectives, were presented:

"to promote fellowship of members"
"to establish and maintain a universal standard of training"
"further the best interests of the nursing profession" [American Society of Superintendents of Training Schools for Nurses, 1985, p. 4].

By 1903, the formal Committee on Education (one of the American Society of Superintendents of Training Schools for Nurses' oldest and most active committees during that time) was established and resulted in the beginning evolution of professional education and training of nurses. The purpose of the Committee on Education was to investigate the methods of teaching and training nurses in schools across the nation, note any changes or advances that took place, and report the findings and general progress of nursing education at each annual meeting of the society (American Society of Superintendents of Training Schools for Nurses, 1905, p. 15).

Adelaide Nutting was chair of the committee. The original committee members were:

- Miss Anna Alline, New York Training School, New York City
- Miss Mary Gilmour, New York Training School, New York City
- Miss Helena McMillan, Presbyterian Hospital, Chicago, Illinois
- Miss Clara Noyes, St. Luke's Hospital, New Bedford, Massachusetts

In the 1905 Annual Report for the American Society of Superintendents of Training School for Nurses, Nutting presented the Committee on Education's report on the work it had accomplished to date. Nutting stated that the committee had met in New York and organized the work by seven main topics that were divided among the committee members:

1. "The Training School.
2. Requirements for Admission and Preliminary Instruction.

3. The General Course of Study or Instruction.
   4. Scholarships, Loan Funds and Tuition Fees.
   5. Salaried Instructors.
   6. Post-Graduate Work.
   7. Training School Libraries" (American Society of
Superintendents of Training Schools for Nurses, 1905, pp. 15–16).

Nutting likewise reported that forms requesting specific information on these seven topics had been sent to five hundred training schools for nursing, and the committee was in the process of tabulating the responses.

In addition to the education of nurses, Nutting wished to provide appropriate preparation of graduate nurses to teach in training schools for nurses. Advanced training for nurses who wished to engage in administration or the education of nurses had become a topic within the Society of Superintendents of Training Schools for Nurses as early as 1896, but there were no programs to prepare nurses for educating nursing students. In 1899, a course in "Hospital Economics" had been established at Teachers College, Columbia University, New York City, and by 1907 the Department of Household Administration was created, with a division titled "Hospital Economics." Nutting was named chair of this newly created division at Teachers College. By 1910, new courses had been added and a special department for the training of nurse instructors was established. As a result, Nutting's goal for an educational institution that would prepare competent nurse educators to teach nursing students had been realized through this program (Columbia University, Teachers College, 1981; Dock, 1912; Stewart, 1919).

The work of the American Society of Superintendents of Training Schools for Nurses continued, and while strides were being made, it was a slow process. Nurse leaders across the United States continued to voice their concerns about a lack of standards in the curricula of nurses' training programs. Although nurse leaders in the core of Appalachia had not been present at the first convention of the American Society of Superintendents of Training Schools for Nurses, they too, were worried about the disorganized conditions in nursing education and practice; they agreed with other nurse leaders throughout the nation and voiced their concerns about the need for clear educational standards in the training of nurses. Lillian White, director of nurses at Knoxville General Hospital from 1902 to 1907, was a strong proponent for

II. Evolution of Nursing Education/Professional Nursing

standardizing nursing education. After leaving Knoxville, she went on to serve as superintendent of nurses at Merritt Hospital, Oakland, California. In 1909, White wrote an article that presented a strong argument in support of improving nursing education with standardization of nursing program curricula:

> Now ... much of the responsibility of establishing a uniform curriculum for our training-schools will fall upon the shoulders of our training-school superintendents.... The young nurse should be carefully watched and trained.... A uniform curriculum will doubtless help along theoretical and practical lines, but I beg of you not to forget the ethical.... We must give to others the benefit of our own experiences.... Just as surgery, medicine, and bacteriology have progressed in the last two decades, so our hospitals have had to meet the resultant demands. Our nurses must be kept abreast of the times ... and it behooves us who are so responsible for ... their success ... to see to it that our methods are what they "ought to be." ... All of our patients cannot go to the large city hospitals and much of the criticism and disparagement to which our small hospitals are subject might be avoided could we train our nurses to properly take charge and manipulate the affairs of these same smaller institutions; for you will all agree with me that they stand for much in their individual localities [White, 1909, pp. 459–461].

Due to the extensive focus on nursing education in the vision and work of the American Society of Superintendents of Training Schools for Nurses, in 1912, the name of that organization was changed to the National League of Nursing Education (NLNE). Isabel Hampton, superintendent of the Nurses Training School at Johns Hopkins Hospital in Baltimore, Maryland, became chair of the newly renamed organization. Members of the group set out to establish their purpose and the foundation of their work, which was to develop and maintain a minimum universal standard of nursing education, to further the best interests of the nursing profession, and to promote fellowship of its members through discussions on nursing subjects, interchange of opinions, meetings, and dissemination of papers. The group members further outlined the objectives of the NLNE:

- Define and maintain minimum standards for training school admission and graduation in schools of nursing throughout the country.
- Assist in furthering all matters pertaining to public health.
- Aid in all measures for public good by cooperating with other bodies: educational, philanthropic, and social.

- Promote through meetings, papers, and discussions, cordial professional relations and fellowship.
- Develop and maintain the highest ideals in the nursing profession (Munson, 1934).

In 1913, the NLNE created a separate Education Committee with the specific purpose of developing a standard curriculum for nurses' training schools across the nation (Nutting, 1923). The committee was made up of the following nurses:

- Adelaide Nutting (chair), Teachers College, New York City
- Isabel Stewart (secretary), Teachers College, New York City
- Ella Crandall, New York City
- Mary Gardner, Providence District Nursing Association, Providence, Rhode Island
- Annie Goodrich, Teachers College, New York City
- Mary Wheeler, Illinois Training School, Chicago, Illinois
- Mary Riddle, Newton Hospital, Newton, Massachusetts
- Elsie Lawler, Johns Hopkins Hospital, Baltimore, Maryland
- Mary Beard, Boston Instructional District Nursing Association, Boston, Massachusetts
- Louise Powell, University Hospital, Minneapolis, Minnesota
- Edna Foley, Chicago, Illinois
- Elizabeth Burgess, State Education Department, Albany, New York
- Mary McKechnie, New York City
- Susan Tracy, Jamaica Plains, Massachusetts

Committee members were from large cities on the East Coast and in the Midwest. While none of the members were from Southern Appalachia, the concerns of nurse educators throughout the entire country were recognized, and the outcome of the National League of Nursing Education's work was germane to the professional education of nurses across the nation, including in the Appalachian region. In unison, the committee members wrote:

> The work of the professional nurse is practically the same in all the states of the union, and it would seem to be perfectly evident that the training which is to guarantee a certain acceptable measure of competence, would need to follow somewhat similar lines, whether the nurse is trained in California or New York, and whether the training is given in a small or a large hospital.... It is becoming clearly evident that if she is to do this effectively, we must revise many of our old ideas about the nurse's training.

II. Evolution of Nursing Education/Professional Nursing

The steady expansion into new and exacting fields of effort is continually revealing to us both the strength and weakness of our methods of training.... It is now recognized that if the sick patient is to have the most skillful and competent kind of nursing care, and if nurses are to keep pace with the advances of modern medicine, they must have something more than a mere deftness in precise manipulations and scattered fragments of scientific knowledge which are all that can usually be given in the scant time allowed by most hospital training schools ... she must have a larger measure of scientific knowledge and she must be more highly trained both in observation and judgement [Committee on Education of the National League of Nursing Education, 1922, pp. 5–6].

It took several years to finalize the work of the committee; by 1917, the committee members had established the first Standard Curriculum for Schools of Nursing, which was published in the same year. The purpose and standards that resulted from the committee's work were articulated in the published Standard Curriculum:

1. "To serve as a guide to training schools struggling to establish good standards of nursing education....
2. To represent to the public and to those who wish to study our work ... what ... we conceive to be an acceptable training for the profession of nursing" (Gray, 1918, p. 791)

The standards established by the committee applied to areas of both the hospital and its nurses' training school:

- General Purpose, Character and Standing of the Hospital
- Form and Functions of Training School Control
- Type and Capacity of the Hospital
- Financial Resources
- Teaching Field (Range, Variety, and Character of Services)
- Conditions of Life and Work for Students (Ratio of Nurses to Patients, Hours of Duty, Housing, and Living Conditions)
- The Administrative and Teaching Staff (Faculty of the School)
- Standards of Entrance to Schools of Nursing
- Standards and Methods of Good Teaching
- Teaching Equipment
- Records
- University Affiliations
- References of Nursing Education and Teaching (Committee on Education of the National League of Nursing Education, 1922, p. 10)

Appalachian Nursing

The proposed course of study included practical instruction as well as theoretical instruction. The committee produced an outline of essential subjects to be taught as part of nurses' training:

- Biological and Physical Sciences
- Anatomy and Physiology; Bacteriology and Chemistry
- Household Science
- Nutrition and Cookery; Diet in Disease; Hospital Housekeeping; Housekeeping Problems of Industrial Families
- Prevention of Disease
- Personal Hygiene and Public Sanitation
- Treatment of Disease
- Drugs and Solutions; Materia Medica and Therapeutics; Massage; Special Therapeutics
- Nursing in Different Forms of Disease
- Elementary Nursing Principles and Methods; Elementary Bandaging; Elements of Pathology; Nursing in Medical, Surgical, and Communicable Diseases; Nursing of Infants and Children; Gynecological, Obstetrical and Orthopedic Nursing; Diseases of the Male Genito-Urinary Tract; Diseases of the Eye, Ear, Nose and Throat; Mental and Nervous Diseases; Occupational, Skin and Venereal Diseases; Operating Room Technique; Emergency Nursing and First Aid; Special Disease Problems
- Social and Professional Subjects
- History of Nursing; Elements of Psychology; Ethics; Survey of the Nursing Field; Professional Problems; Modern Social Conditions
- Special Branches of Nursing
- Introduction to Institutional Work; Private Nursing; Public Health Nursing and Social Service; Laboratory Work (Committee on Education of the National League of Nursing Education, 1922, pp. 3–4)

The committee members further explained that the published standards were not a mandate to adopt; rather, they should be used as a guide for good standing. This original curriculum can be viewed as a beginning effort that, through various iterations and revisions, helped shape and standardize nursing education throughout the entire United States, including the core of Appalachia.

II. Evolution of Nursing Education/Professional Nursing

Nurses' Training Schools and Accreditation

As early as 1918, boards of nursing across the nation used the newly published 1917 NLNE Standard Curriculum as a guide to follow in assessing the quality of the nurses' training schools in their states. The boards' approval was frequently referred to as accreditation. The accreditation was granted by each state's Board of Nurse Examiners, indicating that the training school had met the standards outlined in the 1917 NLNE Standard Curriculum. Training schools that met these standards were listed in 1922 as "Schools Accredited by the State Boards of Nurse Examiners." This state approval can be viewed as a forerunner to the granting of formal NLNE accreditation for nurses' training schools. In 1938, many nurses' training schools across the nation, including in the core of Appalachia, applied for formal accreditation. It became evident that a number of training schools in the core of Appalachia had also followed the standards, thereby meeting the criteria for early accreditation or approval by the state boards of nursing between 1918 and 1922.

Schools of Nursing in the Core of Appalachia Accredited by State Boards of Nurse Examiners in 1922

It is reported that the states also accredited nursing programs as early as 1918; however, no formal NLNE official records have been located for that year. The 1917 NLNE standards were used by the states as an approval process, usually referred to as accreditation. This process was voluntary and initiated by the individual training schools' administrators. In 1922, a number of schools were then granted state accreditation/approval by each state's Board of Nurse Examiners. The criteria used was the NLNE Standard Curriculum set forth in 1917; however, it is not clear how rigorously the criteria were applied. Further, several schools approved or accredited by the states in 1922 closed before the 1938 formal NLNE accreditation process. Many of those training schools that were still in existence by 1938 had maintained their standards since 1922 and earned formal NLNE accreditation.

While most nurse leaders in Southern Appalachia may not have been personally involved in the NLNE committees, they followed the efforts to improve formal nursing education. When the 1917 Standard

Appalachian Nursing

Curriculum was published, nurse leaders in the core of Appalachia were supportive and embraced the idea of applying these standards to hospitals and nurses' training schools in the region. The involvement of these nurse leaders in following the NLNE standards to promote high-quality nursing education in the core of Appalachia was evidenced by the significant number of nurses' training schools in this region that adopted the 1917 curriculum standards and later sought and successfully achieved approval/accreditation by their state Board of Nurse Examiners in 1922.

Nurses' training programs that achieved state Board of Nurse Examiners approval or accreditation in 1922 were located in each Appalachian core state:

Georgia
- Harbin Hospital, Rome

Kentucky
- Paintsville Hospital, Paintsville

North Carolina
- Appalachian Hall Sanitarium, Asheville
- Asheville Mission Hospital, Asheville
- Meriwether Hospital, Asheville
- Clarence Barker Memorial Hospital (Biltmore Hospital), Asheville/Biltmore
- Grace Hospital, Morganton

Tennessee
- Baroness Erlanger Training School for Nurses, Chattanooga
- Highlands Sanitarium, Chattanooga
- Newell & Newell Sanitarium, Chattanooga
- West Ellis Hospital, Chattanooga
- Woolford-Johnson Infirmary, Chattanooga
- Knoxville General Hospital, Knoxville
- Knoxville Private Hospital, Knoxville
- Normal Institute Hospital, Knoxville
- Riverside Hospital, Knoxville

Virginia
- George Ben Johnston (Abingdon Hospital), Abingdon
- Chesapeake and Ohio Hospital, Clifton Forge

II. Evolution of Nursing Education/Professional Nursing

- Jefferson Hospital, Roanoke
- Lewis-Gale Hospital, Roanoke
- Roanoke Hospital, Roanoke
- Shenandoah Hospital, Roanoke

West Virginia
- Beckley Hospital, Beckley
- Bluefield Sanitarium, Bluefield
- St. Luke's Hospital, Bluefield
- City Hospital, Buckhannon
- Charleston General Hospital, Charleston
- Kanawha Valley Hospital, Charleston
- McMillan Hospital, Charleston
- St. Francis Hospital, Charleston
- Mason Hospital, Clarksburg
- St. Mary's Hospital, Clarksburg
- Allegheny Heights Hospital, Davis
- City Hospital, Elkins
- Davis Memorial Hospital, Elkins
- Cook Hospital, Fairmont
- Fairmont Hospital, Fairmont
- Sheltering Arms Hospital, Hansford
- Hinton Hospital, Hinton
- Barnette Hospital (colored), Huntington
- C&O Hospital, Huntington
- Guthrie Hospital, Huntington
- Huntington General Hospital, Huntington
- Kessler-Hatfield Hospital, Huntington
- Hoffman Hospital, Keyser
- Logan Hospital, Logan
- Marlinton Hospital, Marlinton
- Kings Daughters Hospital, Martinsburg
- Martinsburg Hospital, Martinsburg
- McKendree Hospital (Miners' Hospital #2), McKendree
- City Hospital, Morgantown
- Memorial Hospital, Princeton
- Princeton Hospital, Princeton
- McClung Hospital, Richwood
- Sacred Heart Hospital, Richwood

Appalachian Nursing

- Greenbrier Valley Hospital, Ronceverte
- Welch Hospital, Welch (American Nurses Association, Publication Committee, 1922)

Dates are difficult to pin down, due to differences in primary sources and changes in names over time, but based on historical research and triangulation of data, the dates provided are accurate.

Schools of Nursing Accredited by State Boards of Nurse Examiners (1922)

School/Hospital	City	Est.	Beds	Graduates	Full-Time Instructors	Students	Course Length (Months)	Weekly Hours on Duty	Total Graduates	Superintendent of Nurses
GEORGIA										
Harbin Hospital	Rome	1909	N/A	N/A	0	N/A	N/A	N/A	20	N/A
KENTUCKY										
Paintsville Hospital	Paintsville	1920	60	1	3	18	N/A	56	N/A	D. E. Armstrong
NORTH CAROLINA										
Appalachian Hall Sanitarium	Asheville	1917	55	0	2	35	N/A	N/A	2	M. Lowe
Asheville Mission Hospital	Asheville	1896	86	0	5	11	N/A	61	73	F. V. Andrews
Meriwether Hospital	Asheville	1909	43	3	0	15	36	62	42	A. Watt
Clarence Barker Memorial Hospital (Biltmore Hospital)	Biltmore	1900–01	44	2	N/A	16	36	54	28	M. P. Laxton
Grace Hospital	Morganton	1910	30	2	0	7	36	54	14	M. P. Allen

School/Hospital	City	Est.	Beds	Graduates	Full-Time Instructors	Students	Course Length (Months)	Weekly Hours on Duty	Total Graduates	Superintendent of Nurses
TENNESSEE										
Baroness Erlanger Training School for Nurses	Chattanooga	1899	130	6	N/A	48	36	56	176	M. Wayne
Highlands Sanitarium	Chattanooga	N/A	N/A	N/A	N/A	N/A	N/A	N/A	N/A	N/A
Newell & Newell Sanitarium	Chattanooga	1908	N/A	N/A	N/A	N/A	N/A	N/A	N/A	N/A
West Ellis Hospital	Chattanooga	N/A	40	3	N/A	15	36	56	55	M. Renner
Woolford-Johnson Infirmary	Chattanooga	N/A	N/A	N/A	N/A	N/A	N/A	N/A	N/A	N/A
Knoxville General Hospital	Knoxville	1902	N/A	N/A	N/A	N/A	N/A	N/A	N/A	N/A
Normal Institute Hospital	Knoxville	N/A	N/A	N/A	N/A	N/A	N/A	N/A	N/A	N/A
Riverside Hospital	Knoxville	1916	N/A	N/A	N/A	N/A	N/A	N/A	N/A	N/A
VIRGINIA										
George Ben Johnston (Abingdon Hospital)	Abingdon	1912	52	4	N/A	13	36	56	15	K. M. Robertson

School/Hospital	City	Est.	Beds	Graduates	Full-Time Instructors	Students	Course Length (Months)	Weekly Hours on Duty	Total Graduates	Superintendent of Nurses
Chesapeake and Ohio Hospital	Clifton Forge	N/A	85	4	N/A	20	36	56	16	M. Berryman
Jefferson Hospital	Roanoke	N/A	N/A	6	2	25	36	52	27	F. I. Lusby
Lewis-Gale Hospital	Roanoke	1911	50	34	N/A	25	36	56	28	S. V. Thacker
Roanoke Hospital	Roanoke	N/A	29	20	N/A	11	36	58	43	M. A. Edler
Shenandoah Hospital	Roanoke	1916	N/A	N/A	N/A	N/A	N/A	N/A	7	N/A
WEST VIRGINIA										
Beckley Hospital	Beckley	1913	N/A	N/A	N/A	N/A	N/A	N/A	19	N/A
Bluefield Sanitorium	Bluefield	1908	60	2	N/A	N/A	N/A	50	24	L. Halley
St. Luke's Hospital	Bluefield	1907	50	2	2	15	'6	60	3	L. O'Brien
City Hospital	Buckhannon	N/A	N/A	N/A	N/A	N/A	N/A	N/A	N/A	N/A
Charleston General Hospital	Charleston	1898	N/A	N/A	N/A	N/A	N/A		64	N/A
Kanawha Valley Hospital	Charleston	1909	50	2	0	23	N/A	70	20	A. H. Bessler
McMillan Hospital	Charleston	1907	N/A	N/A	N/A	N/A	N/A	N/A	24	N/A
St. Francis Hospital	Charleston	1913	65	6	N/A	0	N/A	63	16	M. Kerwin
Mason Hospital	Clarksburg	1916	42	4	0	12	36	23	26	M. W. Davis

School/Hospital	City	Est.	Beds	Graduates	Full-Time Instructors	Students	Course Length (Months)	Weekly Hours on Duty	Total Graduates	Superintendent of Nurses
St. Mary's Hospital	Clarksburg	1905	125	8	1	35	36	65	74	Sr. M. Aquinas
Allegheny Heights Hospital	Davis	1920		0	0	5	36	N/A	13	E. H. Temple
WEST VIRGINIA										
City Hospital	Elkins	1907	N/A	N/A	N/A	N/A	N/A	N/A	N/A	N/A
Davis Memorial Hospital	Elkins	1903	30	1	N/A	22	N/A	61	37	H. Linn
Cook Hospital	Fairmont	1900–01	N/A	N/A	N/A	N/A	N/A	N/A	96	N/A
Fairmont Hospital (Miners' Hospital #3)	Fairmont	1901	N/A	N/A	N/A	N/A	N/A	N/A	3	N/A
Sheltering Arms Hospital	Hansford	1904	67	3	1	5	36	54	67	H. M. Garrati
Hinton Hospital	Hinton	1902	N/A	2	N/A	14	36	68	46	B. Parker
Barnette Hospital (colored)	Huntington	N/A	30	2	N/A	8	36	42	2	C. C. Barnette
C&O Hospital	Huntington	1915	60	5	N/A	14	36	56	14	E. C. Koch
Guthrie Hospital	Huntington	N/A	N/A	N/A	N/A	N/A	N/A	N/A	N/A	N/A
Huntington General Hospital	Huntington	1910	N/A	N/A	N/A	N/A	N/A	N/A	53	N/A

School/Hospital	City	Est.	Beds	Graduates	Full-Time Instructors	Students	Course Length (Months)	Weekly Hours on Duty	Total Graduates	Superintendent of Nurses
Kessler-Hatfield Hospital	Huntington	1916	N/A	N/A	N/A	N/A	N/A	N/A	21	N/A
Hoffman Hospital	Keyser	1905	25	N/A	N/A	N/A	36	70	26	A. F. Giffin
Logan Hospital	Logan	1917	50	1	N/A	17	36	65	14	M. B. Hennessey
Marlinton Hospital	Marlinton	N/A	N/A	2	0	9	N/A	N/A	N/A	N/A
Kings Daughters Hospital	Martinsburg	1915	50	N/A	N/A	N/A	36	68	7	M. M. Hudson
Martinsburg Hospital	Martinsburg	1906	75	2	N/A	17	36	58	N/A	B. M. Young
McKendree Hospital (Miners' Hospital #2)	McKendree	1901	50	2	N/A	12	36	N/A	20	E. L. Kelleher
City Hospital	Morgantown	1901	35	1	N/A	8	36	84	8	N. D. Brewer
Memorial Hospital	Princeton	1918	35	2	0	10	N/A	63	N/A	A. Withee
Princeton Hospital	Princeton	1912	31	20	0	18	36	63	11	N. Mcintosh Noel
McClung Hospital	Richwood	1905	N/A	N/A	N/A	11	N/A	N/A	186	N/A
Sacred Heart Hospital	Richwood	1917	N/A	N/A	N/A	N/A	N/A	N/A	2	N/A
Greenbrier Valley Hospital	Ronceverte	N/A	N/A	N/A	N/A	N/A	N/A	N/A	N/A	N/A
Welch Hospital	Welch	1913	N/A	N/A	N/A	N/A	N/A	N/A	N/A	N/A

(American Nurses Association, Publication Committee, 1922)

Appalachian Nursing

Although strides had been made since the first Standard Curriculum for Schools of Nursing in 1917, nurse leaders continued to have concerns. In a 1923 speech, Adelaide Nutting remarked about the current state of nursing education:

> What one surveys then in looking back over the developments in nursing is a period of nearly fifty years of almost unrestricted experiment with a system of education in which the school has existed as an integral part of the hospital, created and conducted to serve its needs, with the education of the nurse becoming thereby and inevitably a by-product of her service to the hospital [Nutting, 1923, p. 1028].

Leaders continued to work on the standards, and a revised version of the Standard Curriculum for Schools of Nursing was published in 1927. Examples of a standard curriculum for nurses' training schools in West Virginia set by the NLNE for 1927 and revised in 1937 were published by the West Virginia State Nurses Association. Those standards had been adopted by the West Virginia Board of Nurse Examiners and were illustrative of most training programs throughout the core of Appalachia.

Standard Curriculum Adopted by the West Virginia Board of Nurse Examiners (1927)

Probation and First Year of the Program

Practical Nursing Procedures	Elementary Dietetics
Bandaging	Hygiene and Sanitation
Chemistry	Anatomy and Physiology
Drugs and Solutions	Materia Medica
Ethics and Nursing History	

Intermediate Year in the Program

Dietetic	Anesthesia
Laboratory Diagnosis	Obstetrical Nursing
Bacteriology	Operating Room Technique
Massage	Psychology

Senior Year in the Program

Medical Nursing	Laboratory Diagnosis
Obstetrical Nursing	Nervous and Mental Diseases
Pediatrics	Eye, Ear, Nose and Throat
Advanced Ethics	Special Topics and Review

(Bond, 1957, p. 163)

II. Evolution of Nursing Education/Professional Nursing

From 1934 to 1937, state curriculum committees were organized, in which nurse leaders from each state were appointed as chairs of the state committees to work with the NLNE's Central Curriculum Committee. The core of Appalachia was represented by the state of Tennessee, with Sister Mary Celeste (St. Mary's School of Nursing in Knoxville) as chair, followed later by Elizabeth Newman (Baroness Erlanger Hospital in Chattanooga).

A final version of the standard curriculum, published in 1937, also called for objective measures to determine educational outcomes. In 1938, the NLNE began formal national accreditation for nursing programs across the United States.

Example of the 1937 Standard Curriculum Adopted by the West Virginia Board of Nurse Examiners

First Year of the Program

Elementary Nursing	Anatomy and Physiology
Personal Hygiene	History of Nursing
Ethics	Bacteriology
Materia Medica	Dietetics
Nursing in Surgical Diseases	Medical Nursing
Urinalysis & Pathology	Psychology
Massage	Case Study

Second Year of the Program

Diet in Disease	O.R. Technique
Obstetrics & Gynecology	Nursing in Communicable Disease
Pediatric Nursing	Urology
Orthopedics	Disease of Eye, Ear, Nose and Throat
Skin & Venereal Disease	Elements of Sociology

Third Year of the Program

Mental and Nervous Diseases	Emergency and First Aid
Survey of the Nursing Field	(American Red Cross Text)
Public Health Nursing	Public Hygiene and Sanitation
Review of Nursing Principles and Practice	Oral Surgery

(Bond, 1957, pp. 163–165)

Appalachian Nursing

NATIONAL LEAGUE OF NURSING EDUCATION: FORMAL ACCREDITATION (1938)

There were five training schools of nursing within the core of Appalachia (including a border county—Roanoke) that had been established before 1900 and went on to achieve formal National League of Nursing Education (NLNE) accreditation in 1938. Four of those schools (Asheville Mission Hospital, Asheville, North Carolina; Baroness Erlanger Hospital, Chattanooga, Tennessee; Roanoke Hospital, Roanoke, Virginia; and Charleston General Hospital, Charleston, West Virginia) had also received State Board of Nurse Examiners accreditation/approval in 1922. It is not clear whether Berea College actually attempted approval/accreditation in 1922.

Kentucky
- Berea College Training School for Nurses (founded 1898), Berea

North Carolina
- Asheville Mission Hospital Training School for Nurses (founded 1896), Asheville (also accredited/approved by the North Carolina State Board of Nurse Examiners in 1922)

Tennessee
- Baroness Erlanger Training School for Nurses (founded 1899), Chattanooga (also accredited/approved by the Tennessee State Board of Nurse Examiners in 1922)

Virginia
- Roanoke Hospital (founded 1899), Roanoke (border county of Appalachian core; also accredited/approved by the Virginia State Board of Nurse Examiners in 1918 and 1922)

West Virginia
- Charleston General Hospital Training School for Nurses (founded 1898), Charleston (also accredited/approved by the West Virginia State Board of Nurse Examiners in 1938)

The following training schools for nurses in the core of Appalachia likewise received formal accreditation by the National League of Nursing Education in 1938. The NLNE report was published in 1939.

North Carolina
- Highland Hospital (founded 1904), Asheville

II. Evolution of Nursing Education/Professional Nursing

- Biltmore Hospital (formerly Clarence Barker Memorial Hospital), Asheville accredited/approved by the North Carolina State Board of Nurse Examiners in 1922)
- Grace Hospital (founded 1924), Banner Elk
- Mountain Sanitarium and Hospital (founded 1929), Fletcher
- Grace Hospital (founded 1910), Morganton (also accredited/approved by the North Carolina State Board of Nurse Examiners in 1922)

Tennessee
- Newell & Newell Sanitarium (founded 1908), Chattanooga (also accredited/approved by the Tennessee State Board of Nurse Examiners in 1922)
- Greenville Sanitarium Training School for Nurses, Greenville
- Takoma Hospital Training school for Nurses, Greeneville
- Appalachian (previously Memorial) Hospital Training School for Nurses (founded 1902), Johnson City
- Parker-Budd Clinic (founded 1935), Johnson City
- Fort Sanders Hospital Training School for Nurses (founded 1920), Knoxville
- Howard Henderson Hospital Training School for Nurses (founded 1927), Knoxville
- Knoxville General Hospital (founded 1902), Knoxville (also accredited/approved by the Tennessee State Board of Nurse Examiners in 1922)
- St. Mary's Hospital Training School for Nurses (founded 1930), Knoxville

Virginia
- George Ben Johnston Memorial Hospital (founded 1912), Abingdon (also accredited/approved by the Virginia State Board of Nurse Examiners in 1922)
- Chesapeake and Ohio Hospital (founded 1917), Clifton Forge (also accredited/approved by the Virginia State Board of Nurse Examiners in 1922)
- Lewis-Gale Hospital (founded 1911), Roanoke (Appalachia core border county; also accredited/approved by the Virginia State Board of Nurse Examiners in 1922)
- Jefferson Hospital (founded 1914), Roanoke (Appalachia core

border county; also accredited/approved by the Virginia State Board of Nurse Examiners in 1922)
- Catawba Sanatorium (founded 1910), Roanoke/Catawba

West Virginia
- Raleigh General Hospital (founded 1928), Beckley
- St. Luke's Hospital (founded 1907), Bluefield (also accredited/approved by the West Virginia State Board of Nurse Examiners in 1922)
- Kanawha Valley Hospital (founded 1909), Charleston (also accredited/approved by the West Virginia State Board of Nurse Examiners in 1922)
- McMillan Hospital (founded 1907), Charleston (also accredited/approved by the West Virginia State Board of Nurse Examiners in 1922)
- Mountain State Hospital (founded 1921), Charleston
- St. Francis Hospital (founded 1913), Clarksburg (also accredited/approved by the West Virginia State Board of Nurse Examiners in 1922)
- St. Mary's Hospital (founded 1905), Clarksburg (also accredited/approved by the West Virginia State Board of Nurse Examiners in 1922)
- City Hospital (founded 1907), Elkins (also accredited/approved by the West Virginia State Board of Nurse Examiners in 1922)
- Davis Memorial Hospital (founded 1903), Elkins (also accredited/approved by the West Virginia State Board of Nurse Examiners in 1922)
- Cook Hospital (founded ca. 1900–01), Fairmont (also accredited/approved by the West Virginia State Board of Nurse Examiners in 1922)
- *Fairmont Emergency Hospital (founded 1907), Fairmont (also accredited/approved by the West Virginia State Board of Nurse Examiners in 1922)
- Hinton Hospital (founded 1902), Hinton
- Huntington Memorial Hospital (founded Huntington General and Williamson hospitals in 1910; merged with Huntington Memorial ca. 1921), Huntington (also accredited/approved by the West Virginia State Board of Nurse Examiners in 1922)

II. Evolution of Nursing Education/Professional Nursing

- St. Mary's Hospital (founded 1923), Huntington
- McKendree Hospital* (founded 1901), McKendree (also accredited/approved by the West Virginia State Board of Nurse Examiners in 1922)
- Laird Memorial Hospital (originally Coal Valley Hospital; founded 1918), Montgomery
- City Hospital (founded 1912), Morgantown (also accredited/approved by the West Virginia State Board of Nurse Examiners in 1922)
- Greenbrier Valley Hospital (founded 1921), Ronceverte (also accredited/approved by the West Virginia State Board of Nurse Examiners in 1922)
- Welch Hospital* (founded 1914), Welch (also accredited/approved by the West Virginia State Board of Nurse Examiners in 1922)

also known as Miners' Hospitals

In 1938, West Virginia claimed the largest number of NLNE-accredited nurses' training programs in the core of Appalachia (20), followed by Tennessee (10) (National League of Nursing Education, 1939).

The number of training schools in the core of Appalachia earning formal NLNE accreditation in 1938 and/or those earning 1922 state Board of Nurse Examiners' approval suggests that although there were few nurses in the core of Appalachia who were active members of any formal NLNE committees, the emphasis on quality of nursing education had apparently been considered paramount; the early education standards were followed by nursing administrators in a significant number of training schools, which ultimately had a positive impact on many of the nurses' training schools in Appalachia.

1938–39 NLNE Accreditation Hospitals

School/Hospital	City	Est.	Beds	Students	Course Length (Months)	Weekly Hours on Duty	Full-Time Instructors	Affiliation w/ Community Health Agency	School Director
KENTUCKY									
Berea College	Berea	1898	130	37	36	42	1	Yes	N. Cox Hare
NORTH CAROLINA									
Asheville Mission	Asheville	1896	130	49	36	58	1	No	A. M. Perry
Biltmore Hospital (Clarence Barker Memorial)	Asheville/ Biltmore	1900–01	62	32	36	54	1	No	R. Hampton
Highland Hospital	Asheville	1904	85	22	36	56	1	No	G. Sykes
Grace Hospital	Banner Elk	1924	60	25	36	56	1	No	R. B. Reynolds
Mountain Sanitarium and Hospital	Fletcher	1929	60	23	36	50	N/A	No	E. Pearson
Grace Hospital	Morganton	1910	92	18	36	N/A	1	Yes	M. Maddrey
TENNESSEE									
Baroness Erlanger Training School for Nurses	Chattanooga	1899	250	108	36	52.5	2	No	S. M. Hocks
Newell & Newell Sanitarium	Chattanooga	1908	65	33	36	57	0	No	B.G. Bearden

School/Hospital	City	Est.	Beds	Students	Course Length (Months)	Weekly Hours on Duty	Full-Time Instructor	Affiliation w/ Community Health Agency	School Director
Greeneville Sanitarium and Hospital	Greeneville		N/A	N/A	N/A	N/A	N/A	N/A	N/A
Takoma Hospital and Sanitarium	Greeneville		N/A	N/A	N/A	N/A	N/A	N/A	N/A
Appalachian (Memorial) Hospital	Johnson City	1902	75	26	36	32–35	1	No	E. M. Doty
Parker-Budd Clinic	Johnson City	1935	22	6	36	42	1	No	C. J. Budd, MD
Howard Henderson Hospital	Knoxville	1927	44	16	36	42	1	No	V. Heritage
Fort Sanders Hospital	Knoxville	1920	175	68	36	52	2	No	E. Killeffer
Knoxville General Hospital	Knoxville	1902	312	108	36	56	1	No	L. Humphreys Greene
St. Mary's Hospital	Knoxville	1930	75	35	36	42	N/A	No	Sr. Mary Celeste
VIRGINIA									
George Ben Johnston Memorial Hospital	Abingdon	1912	65	22	36	52	1	Yes	N. E. Seay
Chesapeake and Ohio Hospital	Clifton Forge	1917	148	36–42	36	52	1	No	P. Pope
Jefferson Hospital	Roanoke	1914	110	41	36	42	1	No	B. B. Sumpter
Lewis-Gale Hospital	Roanoke	1911	132	63	36	54	1	No	S. V. Thacker
Roanoke Hospital	Roanoke	1899	110	42	36	48	1	No	M. Lowe
Catawba Sanatorium	Roanoke	1910	340	23	36	N/A	1	No	M. E. Ewald

School/Hospital	City	Est.	Beds	Students	Course Length (Months)	Weekly Hours on Duty	Full-Time Instructors	Affiliation w/ Community Health Agency	School Director
WEST VIRGINIA									
Raleigh General Hospital	Beckley	1928	74	22	36	56	1	No	M. E. Taliaferro
St. Luke's Hospital	Bluefield	1907	83	39	36	42	2	No	G. Hughes
Charleston General Hospital Training School for Nurses	Charleston	1898	250	83	36	42	2	No	A. C. Corbitt
Kanawha Valley	Charleston	1909	130	50	36	46	1	No	A. H. Bessier
McMillan Hospital	Charleston	1907	100	30	36	52	1	No	S. Hamilton
Mountain State Hospital	Charleston	1921	87	25	36	54	1	No	Sr. Mary de Lourdes
St. Francis Hospital	Charleston	1913	104	34	36	48	1	No	Sr. M. Virginia
St. Mary's Hospital	Clarksburg	1905	165	52	36	48	1	No	M. J. Pickrell
City Hospital	Elkins	1907	71	18	36	56	0	No	G. L. Rosencrance
Davis Memorial	Elkins	1903	125	30	36	N/A	1	No	O. A. Campion
Cook/Fairmont General Hospital	Fairmont	1902	120	30	36	44	1	Yes	M. Robertson
Fairmont Emergency Hospital	Fairmont	1907	75	25	36	48	1	No	J. L. Price
Hinton Hospital	Hinton	1902	75	21	36	45	1	No	D.K Howard

School/Hospital	City	Est.	Beds	Students	Course Length (Months)	Weekly Hours on Duty	Full-Time Instructors	Affiliation w/ Community Health Agency	School Director
Huntington Memorial Hospital	Huntington	1904	135	32	36	56	1	No	M. Robertson
St. Mary's Hospital	Huntington	1923	250	68	36	46	2	Yes	Sr. M. Pia
McKendree Emergency Hospital	McKendree	1901	75	68	36	51	0	No	J. E. Weeks
Coal Valley/Laird Memorial Hospital	Montgomery	1918	135	51	36	56	1	No	M. E. Meredith
City Hospital	Morgantown	1912	74	20	36	N/A	1	No	J. B. Robinson
Greenbrier Valley	Ronceverte	1921	90	12	36	49	1	No	L. M. Harless
Welch Hospital	Welch	1914	N/A	N/A	N/A	N/A	N/A	N/A	N/A

(*National League of Nursing Education, 1939*)

Appalachian Nursing

A Cross Section of Nurses' Training Schools in the Core of Appalachia That Achieved 1922 State Board of Nurse Examiners' Accreditation, NLNE 1938 Formal Accreditation, or Both

Note: This is not an exclusive list, but rather a portion of the training schools that met accreditation requirements.

Georgia Nurses' Training Schools

Harbin Hospital Training School for Nurses, Rome, Georgia

Until the establishment in 1908 of Harbin Hospital in Rome (Floyd County), Georgia, there were no known hospital nurses' training schools in Georgia's Appalachian core counties during the early twentieth century. Most of the nurses' training schools in the state had been established in areas outside the core of Appalachia. Harbin Hospital was founded by Drs. R.M. and W.P. Harbin, brothers who graduated from Bellevue Hospital Medical College in 1897. The original hospital had 12 beds and was located in a residence in Rome, Georgia. The doctors added a nurses' training program, and in 1909 the Harbin Hospital Training School for Nurses was established (American Nurses Association, 1922). By 1919, a new four-story hospital was constructed, offering 75 beds. In 1920, three more stories were added, and the hospital was considered state of the art, with all modern conveniences. The original hospital was converted to a dormitory for the nurses' training program.

The hospital was recognized by the American College of Surgeons in 1921 as one of the four hospitals in Georgia that met the medical board's standards of excellence. On Hospital Day in May of that same year, Harbin Hospital had 29 nurses and was opened to visitors. Nurses conducted tours, escorting the visitors through patients' rooms, operating suites, the laboratory, and x-ray rooms.

In 1922, the Harbin Hospital nurses' training program was included with 32 other training schools in the state of Georgia as having met the criteria set forth in 1917 by the National League for Nursing Education and achieved Georgia's Board of Nurse Examiners' accreditation for the state that year.

Dr. R.M. Harbin, one of the brothers who had established the hospital, presented a paper in 1923 to the Floyd County Medical Society and Rome Georgia Nursing Association, in which he characterized the

II. Evolution of Nursing Education/Professional Nursing

profession of nursing as an opportunity. Harbin began his presentation referring to nursing as "one of the ennobling profession—ennobling in that it gives opportunity for the display of those higher altruistic ideals that are foreign to so many vocations" (Harbin, 1923, p. 96), suggesting that nursing also brought a human touch to patients. He went on to say:

> Nursing is a true profession—a career for the attainment for those higher ideals that are offered to women, second only to that of the Christian religion.... Of all careers open to women, nursing to my mind, is most remunerative and it has not that monotonous grind that applies to office or shop work every day in the week measured off by the clock [Harbin, 1923, p. 97].

It should be noted that during the early years of Harbin Hospital's training school for nurses, the women's suffrage movement was taking place in the United States, and women were finally granted the right to vote in 1919. Although Harbin was somewhat complimentary about the role of nurses in his 1923 presentation, he concluded his presentation with comments reflecting the long-standing views of women's role in society that were still prevalent during that time: "Nurses can make money and do save money, but many mismanage well earned gains. Women as a rule do not value money as much as do men" (Harbin, 1923, p. 97).

Harbin also provided his view on nurses and marriage: "I am not prepared to give statistics on this, but I am prepared to believe that nurses who do get married make better and more successful marriages than they would have done if they had not been nurses" (Harbin, 1923, p. 97).

Although the training school met requirements for state accreditation in 1922, it was not formally accredited by the NLNE in 1938. In 1948, when Harbin Hospital was converted to a medical clinic, patients were seen on an outpatient basis, and the nurses' training school closed (Harbin Clinic, n.d.).

Kentucky Nurses' Training Schools

Berea Hospital

Berea College was founded by abolitionist John Fee in 1855 as the first racially integrated college in the South. In 1898, Berea Hospital was established by the college to care for its students. Soon after the hospital was established, a nurses' training department was created. Potential nursing students had to be at least 18 years old and in good health, with above-average strength and energy validated by a physician's letter. The applicant also had to be of good moral character (validated by a church minister). Students were likewise required to demonstrate competence in reading, writing, and math. Those students who were provisionally accepted into the program had a three-month probation period in which they were employed at the hospital, observing the experienced nurses and learning how to care for the patients. Once the potential students passed the probation period, they were accepted into the full-time nursing program. The original program was two years long; however, the Kentucky state registration act of 1916 required nurses' training programs to be three years in length before a graduate nurse could become registered. William Frost, president of Berea College at this time, was hoping to prepare nurses to take care of people in the mountains who could not afford highly trained nurses, which was considered to be following the mission of the college. He also resisted a three-year program, stating, "We feel that it would not be useful for the mountain region for us to prepare nurses so highly trained as this. They would insist upon high pay and be lost for mountain service" (Dent, 2020).

Once Frost left his position at Berea College in 1920, the college expanded the nursing program to three years by 1921. The program also included a nine-month experience in a Louisville hospital, but later it switched to a hospital in Cincinnati, Ohio, so the students would have the benefit of working with patients exhibiting a variety of diseases (an opportunity not always available at Berea). The three-year program allowed students to meet the requirements needed to take the state exam to become registered nurses. In 1925, the department name was changed to the School of Nursing. Berea was also one of the many nursing schools that offered the cadet nurse program approved in 1943 by the Division of Nurses of the U.S. Public Health Service. The three-year nurses' training program continued until 1956, when it was increased to a four-year baccalaureate degree program (Dent, 2020).

Paintsville Hospital

The Paintsville Hospital in Johnson County, Kentucky (a coal mining area), opened in November 1920 with 25 beds. In a history of the hospital, Dr. Paul B. Hall wrote that the establishment of a hospital in Paintsville originated with Dr. Ernest Archer, who, along with Dr. J.H. Holbrook and Dr. James Sparks, received financial support through the North East Coal Company and several other individuals. The hospital's

II. Evolution of Nursing Education/Professional Nursing

first superintendent was nurse Malissa Osborne. Shortly after the hospital was established, a nurses' training school was created through a charter granted by the Kentucky State Nurses' Association. By 1922, the school had two graduates and one instructor, and it was accredited by Kentucky's Board of Nurse Examiners. The nurses' training school, however, closed several years later when it was decided there was an overabundance of registered nurses in the state of Kentucky (Hall, 2009).

North Carolina Nurses' Training Schools

Grace Hospital, Banner Elk

As in other communities in the core of Appalachia, Banner Elk was a small community located in the remote western North Carolina mountains. Access to a doctor or hospital was limited, and travel to the closest hospital meant a trip over rough mountainous terrain. During the winter, roads were impassable, so when residents of the community became ill, they relied on home remedies.

In 1895, the Concord Presbytery sent Edgar Tufts, a seminary student, to establish a church in Banner Elk. Beyond fulfilling his religious mission, Tufts also found that the community was limited in educational opportunities and would benefit from having a school. With the assistance of benefactor Susanna Lees and teacher Elizabeth McRae, the Lees-McRae Institute was established in 1907. In addition to education, the community of Banner Elk was in need of medical care. In 1908, as a way to provide the much-needed healthcare for Banner Elk, the presbytery made arrangements to build a doctor's residence and office, two patient rooms, an operating room and a laboratory. A retired medical missionary physician was recruited to serve the community. The physician stayed for a couple of years and was replaced by another practitioner, Dr. C.W. Tate, who had graduated from the University of Tennessee Medical College. It was common for patients to be treated at home unless they required surgery. However, by 1923, the need for more hospital space to care for patients became critical. With donated funds, a new hospital was built in 1924, and that same year a formal training school for nurses was established.

The training program for nurses was three years in length, with a four-month probationary period during the first year. Students were required to have a high school diploma for admission to the school.

Appalachian Nursing

There was a preference for applicants to be Christian. The school was operated under a theological umbrella with a strict code of conduct. Most of the lectures were provided by the superintendent of nurses. Nursing students were forbidden to speak to boys (even those who attended the local Lees-McRae College). Other rules that nursing students had to follow during their training and work at the hospital included the following:

- When on duty, nurses were to rise and remain standing while talking to doctors, superintendents, or their assistants.
- Nurses were not allowed to accept or receive personal services from their patients (i.e., running errands, sewing, etc.).
- Nurses were not to go off duty without first reporting to the charge nurse.
- Nurses could not consult the doctor without first reporting to the superintendent.
- Nurses could not take drugs for their own use or prescribe or give out drugs to another nurse.
- Nurses could not accept visitors while on duty or in the wards.
- When off duty, nurses could not return to the wards, have visitors in their rooms, or escort visitors through the building without first asking the superintendent.
- A nurse could not return to her room without first asking permission from the charge nurse.
- Nurses could not go shopping or visiting in uniform.
- Nurses were to wear a full uniform while on duty. Shoes were to be noiseless. Uniforms were inspected on the first day of every month.
- All nurses were to be in their rooms by 10:00 p.m.; lights went out at 10:30 p.m.
- One late permit was allowed each week. During the months of training, student nurses were allowed one evening off per week. If they left the building after 7:00 p.m. or stayed out later, there was a book where they signed in, in addition to notifying the superintendent.
- Night nurses were to be in bed by 10:00 p.m. and up by 5:00 a.m.
- Student rooms were inspected weekly.
- Nurses were required to clean their own rooms on Friday or Saturday.

II. Evolution of Nursing Education/Professional Nursing

- Nurses could not visit the kitchen other than at their mealtime (Pollitt & Moore 1992).

Tennessee Nurses' Training Schools

Baroness Erlanger Training School for Nurses, Chattanooga

Chattanooga's Training School for Nurses at Baroness Erlanger Hospital opened in 1899 with Anna Hand as the first director of nursing education. By 1901, the first class of five nursing students graduated: Daisy Duncan, Belle George, Jessie Rose, Annie Thomas, and Margaret Thompson.

Jessie Rose, a 1901 graduate, became the director of nursing education at Baroness Erlanger in 1902. Katherine Farmer, a 1904 graduate, became the first visiting nurse for Metropolitan Life in Chattanooga, Tennessee, and 1914 graduate Helen Burt served during World War I in the Army Nurse Corps. In 1913, the nurses' training program was increased from two to three years. Requirements for 1919 admission to the nurses' training program included a minimum of one year of high school, a statement from a minister testifying to the applicant's moral character, and statements from a dentist and doctor verifying the prospective student's health. The student's day included three to four hours of classroom instruction and seven to eight hours working in a ward or a laboratory. Classroom topics included anatomy, bandages, "nervous" diseases, obstetrics and gynecology (Poole & Sawyer, 1993).

Memorial Hospital, Johnson City

By 1903, Johnson City, Tennessee, was home to a military hospital on the Mountain Home Military Reservation (now the Veterans Administration Campus), where it served military veterans. However, the community lacked a hospital for all of its residents. In addition, there was no formal nurses' training available in northeast Tennessee. Six local physicians recognized the need for a community hospital and, in 1911, established Memorial Hospital, the first in a progression of three hospitals that included schools of nursing and were forerunners of East Tennessee State University's College of Nursing. The new hospital began with 10 beds in a small wooden duplex and offered a training school for nurses (Stahl, 1989).

Amelia Young, a 1911 graduate of Lincoln Memorial Hospital's Training School for Nurses in Knoxville, Tennessee, was hired as the first superintendent and director of the nurses' training school at the newly established hospital. The school opened with two student nurse probationers, Orlena Elizabeth Morris and Lucille Andis. The nursing students worked at the hospital during the day and attended physician lectures at night. In 1912, Morris became the first graduate of Memorial Hospital Training School for Nurses, followed by Andis in 1913.

During this time, nursing in the Appalachian region was not considered a respected profession. A grandniece of 1912 graduate Orlena Morris recalled a conversation about nursing that she had with her great-aunt:

> Aunt Lena once told me that she had been the first nursing graduate of Memorial Hospital School of Nursing. Her family was scandalized over the possibility that her professional duties might require her to see and/or touch male patients in a state of partial or full undress. My spunky old aunt dismissed those fears with one snort! Lena had a backbone of steel and her being a nurse was one of the most important things in her life [Reel, personal conversation, Johnson City, Tennessee, June 23, 2014].

There were a number of superintendents who followed the resignation of Amelia Young: Lulu Hodge in 1911, Lena Singleton in 1914, Amanda Jarvis in 1917, and Marie Smith in 1919. Memorial Hospital and its nurses' training school continued to serve the community until 1921, but the need for expanded hospital space resulted in the construction of a larger facility that was renamed Appalachian Hospital. Ida Garrett, graduate of Knoxville General Hospital, became the superintendent of nurses at the new Appalachian Hospital.

By that time the nursing program had expanded from one to three years. Nursing students spent 60 hours per week in the program (56 hours in hospital work and 4 hours per week in classroom lectures conducted at night). After a series of nurse superintendents, Vesta Swartz from the University of Maryland was hired as superintendent in 1941. By 1943, through Swartz's efforts, Appalachian Hospital and East Tennessee State College reached an agreement in which Appalachian Hospital nursing students could take courses in psychology, English, and chemistry for credit at the college.

Virginia Nurses' Training Schools

George Ben Johnston Memorial School of Nursing, Abingdon

The George Ben Johnston Hospital started out in 1905 as Abingdon Hospital, a small facility established for the community by Dr. E.T.

II. Evolution of Nursing Education/Professional Nursing

Brady of Abingdon, Virginia, but, due to lack of patients, it closed in June 1910. That summer Drs. George Ben Johnston (of southwest Virginia) and A. M Willis of the Johnston-Willis Sanatorium in Richmond, Virginia, became aware of the Abingdon community's need, and they bought a controlling interest in the hospital. The hospital reopened in the fall of that same year but had no staff. At that point, in order to staff the newly opened hospital, the doctors resorted to "borrowing" student nurses from a hospital in Richmond. By 1912, a training school for nurses had been established at the hospital. The first superintendent of nurses was Mamie Rice. In 1914, the first nurses to graduate from Ben Johnston Hospital Training School for Nurses were Miss Katy Robertson and Miss Henderson, transfers from the Johnston-Willis Sanatorium in 1913. In 1915, Lou Willa Honaker became the first graduate of the full nursing program at Ben Johnston Hospital, and, in 1916, Katy Robertson became the superintendent. This institution was considered

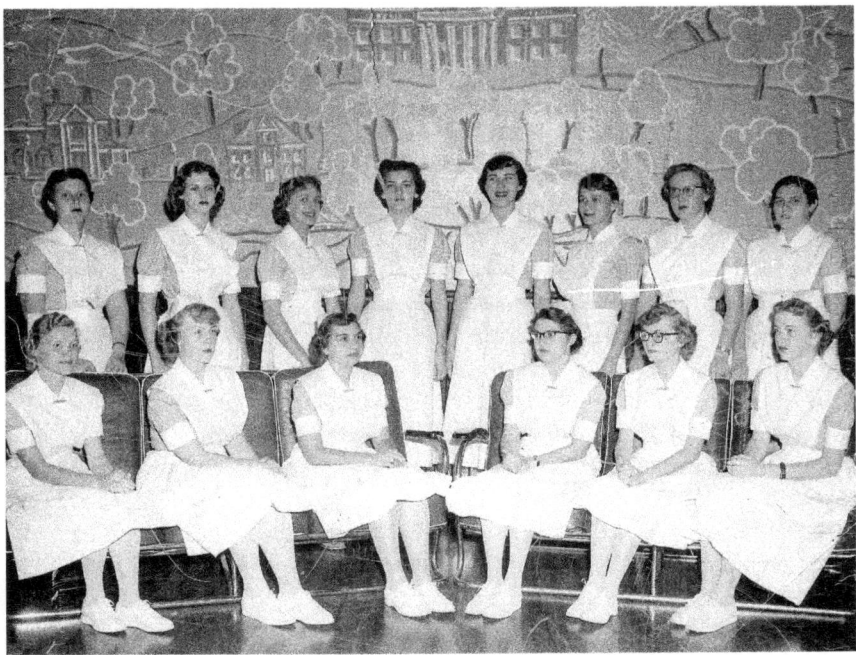

Evelyn Price Jones (third from left, back row) at the 1957 graduation of the BSN class, Emory & Henry College (courtesy Evelyn Price Jones).

one of the first known formal training schools for nurses in southwest Virginia (Stephenson, 1947).

Eventually the name of George Ben Johnston Hospital was changed to Johnston Memorial Hospital, and, during the 1950s, the school of nursing became a diploma program. An affiliation was developed between Emory & Henry College and the hospital, so that Johnston Memorial Hospital nursing students could earn a four-year baccalaureate degree. One graduate of this program was Evelyn Price Jones, who enrolled in the school of nursing and opted for the newly created baccalaureate in nursing degree. She described the first years of her program as being primarily pre-clinical courses taken at Emory & Henry College; the last two years of clinical work were completed at the Johnston Memorial Hospital School of Nursing. Price Jones graduated with 13 other nursing students who had also opted for the BSN program (E. Price Jones, personal interview, April 29, 2020).

West Virginia Nurses' Training Schools

Cook/Fairmont General Hospital, Fairmont

Cook Hospital was founded around 1900–01, and the training school for nurses was established in 1900. The first class of five women graduated in 1902. One nurse who had completed her training at Cook Hospital in 1923 recalled student nurses having a variety of hospital duties that included working in the laundry and scrubbing the floors. They worked twelve hours a day, seven days a week, and were also responsible for cooking special meals to meet patients' dietary requirements. When students were assigned to the operating room, they had to be in the room by 4:30 in the morning and, in preparation for the day, build fires to create pressure for the autoclave. Students also had to pre–hand wash the soiled laundry from surgeries before sending it to the main laundry. Nursing students wore starched, white, long-sleeved, floor-length uniforms. The cost of attending the training school was low and students were provided with room and board, which, for many, was a financial benefit. One nurse who completed her training in 1934 shared that students applying to the training school during the 1930s had requirements similar to those of earlier graduates. Doctors provided most of the lectures at the hospital, and students were required to have their own instruments, including syringes and bandage scissors. They were given three weeks' vacation and could go home during that time. The graduate also shared that nurses on duty at the hospital were

II. Evolution of Nursing Education/Professional Nursing

responsible for everything when the doctors were not in the building. She recalled that they cared for a lot of coal miners. The hospital did not have an emergency department, and funeral homes provided ambulances to transport patients to the hospital. When injuries happened in the mines, the miners were brought to a patient room where the nurses would care for them until the doctors arrived. Many times the surgeons brought their own equipment; for any other items needed, they called the local hardware stores. There were no pharmacists on duty, so private pharmacists in the area were called when there was a question (Bond, 1957).

The training school for nurses was accredited by the state Board of Nurse Examiners in 1922 and achieved national accreditation by the NLNE in 1938. The name Cook Hospital was changed to Fairmont Hospital in 1939, which became Fairmont General Hospital in 1940. In 1943, the nursing school became affiliated with Fairmont State College (Alvarez, 1992; American Nurses Association, Publication Committee, 1922).

Charleston General Hospital Training School for Nurses (Originally Thomas' Hospital Training School for Nurses)

Charleston General Hospital, beginning its existence in the late 1880s as Thomas's Hospital, underwent a number of name changes. In 1898, a training school for nurses was established. The training school was discontinued in 1905 and then reorganized in 1922, with the first class graduating in 1926. In that same year, Miss Mae Fye was listed as director, followed by Miss Alma Corbitt in 1929. Corbitt retired from active nursing on February 28, 1957, and was succeeded by Mrs. Mary S. Turner. The nurses' training school received national accreditation in 1938 and maintained accreditation at least through 1957, if not later. As a participant in the cadet nurse program, the training school also had an affiliation with Morris Harvey College and clinical psychiatry with Chestnut Lodge of Rockville, Maryland (Bond, 1957).

Goldmark Report and University-Level Nursing Education

As with the 1910 Flexner Report (an evaluation of medical education in schools throughout the United States), there was a concerted effort to improve the education of nurses, and in 1918 the Rockefeller Foundation funded the Committee for the Study of Nursing Education to evaluate public health nursing and nursing education. Based on her background in social research, Josephine Goldmark was appointed secretary of the committee to organize the investigation. The 1923 written committee report, "Nursing and Nursing Education in the United States," became commonly known as the Goldmark Report. The committee was formed in 1919 and included the following nurse leaders, physicians, and public health leaders:

- Mary Beard, Boston (nursing)
- Dr. Herman Biggs, New York (medicine/public health)
- Annie Goodrich, New York (nursing)
- Adelaide Nutting, New York (nursing)
- Lillian Wald, New York (nursing)
- Dr. William Welch, Baltimore (medicine)
- Professor C.E.A. Winslow, New Haven (public health)

Although the committee was originally charged with evaluating the quality of public health nursing education, its mission soon expanded to include the overall general education and training of nurses across the nation. Approximately 1,800 training schools for nurses were surveyed, with 23 schools selected to be studied in detail. Although no nurse leaders in the core of Appalachia were personally involved in the Goldmark study, nor were any schools of nursing in the core of Appalachia clearly identified, the resulting report had a significant impact on nursing education that ultimately included the core of Appalachia and addressed the general and public health education of nurses in the region.

The study resulted in noteworthy findings, including a reference to rural nursing that was geographically representative of nursing in the core of Appalachia. The findings indicated differences among rural nursing, nursing in small towns, and nursing in larger cities across the United States. The committee members found that small towns had advantages similar to those observed in large cities because of the close proximity of patients to one another and ready access to medical facilities and resources, including hospitals, health agencies, and other health-related resources. Rural nurses, however, experienced challenges specific to nursing in isolated regions, including the core of Appalachia, where nurses had limited access to resources such as hospitals, dispensaries, and health-related agencies. Since distances between patients in small towns and cities were short, a nurse could make more home visits in one day and reach her patients in a timely fashion. In contrast, the rural visiting or public health nurse had to negotiate mountainous terrain and nonexistent or impassible roads, where they had to walk or

II. Evolution of Nursing Education/Professional Nursing

ride horseback to see their patients. The rural nurse was frequently the only nurse for the county or region, forced to work singlehanded without necessary health-related resources or access to a local physician.

Other findings from the Goldmark investigation included a number of issues in nursing education that validated the ongoing concerns of nurse leaders:

- In hospitals, the needs of patients took precedence over the need for student education.
- There was insufficient time for nursing students to study.
- There was an excessive length of time when students were on duty in the hospital.
- Students' classes were frequently held in the evenings after long hours on duty.
- There was a lack of qualified teachers.
- Most training school programs failed to include psychology, public health, and social service in their curricula.

Recommendations from the report included the following points:

- Nurses' training schools needed to reorganize.
- Graduation from high school should be required for admission to any nurses' training school.
- Students needed a preliminary term in basic sciences and elementary nursing.
- Superintendents, supervisors, and nursing instructors should have postgraduate training (Committee for the Study of Nursing Education, 1923).

One of the most significant results of the survey was the need and sound rationale for connecting future nurses' training with college education. Yale University followed that recommendation and, in 1924, established a baccalaureate degree in the science of nursing that included nursing education in a separate university department outside the hospital. Following Yale, collegiate nursing programs began to grow in the larger cities across the nation, but they were slow to develop in the core of Appalachia until the middle of the twentieth century.

A partnership between Appalachian Hospital and East Tennessee State College in Johnson City, Tennessee, was a later example of following the Goldmark Report recommendations. Incorporating university-level education into the Appalachian Hospital nursing program resulted in the establishment of a baccalaureate in nursing degree program at East Tennessee State College in 1954.

Nurse leaders in the Appalachian region had also been discussing nursing education issues and the importance of incorporating university-level education into hospital-based nursing programs. They agreed with the early recommendations from the Goldmark Report of providing early access to college-level education for nursing students. In 1941, Vesta Swartz, an assistant superintendent of nurses at the School of Nursing in Baltimore, Maryland, was hired as the superintendent of Appalachian Hospital's nurses' training program. Swartz was a proponent of the Goldmark Report and felt strongly about the improvement of nurses' training and college-level education for nurses. She agreed that the service needs of a hospital should not override the educational needs of the student nurse and that the graduate nurse should have a college education component in his or her training program. Much of Swartz's time and effort in Johnson City was spent on improving nursing education at Appalachian (later named Memorial) Hospital School of Nursing while also expanding the students' training to include college-level courses. In 1943, Swartz approached the administration of East Tennessee State College (ETSC) with the suggestion of establishing a formal affiliation between Appalachian Hospital School of Nursing and ETSC. The plan was for Appalachian Hospital nursing students to enroll at ETSC in general education courses while attending the hospital's training program. A formal partnership emerged between Appalachian Hospital School of Nursing and ETSC in which nursing students received their first nine months of coursework at ETSC. The Appalachian Hospital nursing students were enrolled for three quarters at ETSC and took the following courses: physiology, psychology, sociology, principles of nursing, English, microbiology, chemistry, nutrition, and cooking.

In 1951, Appalachian Hospital became Memorial Hospital, and over several years Swartz continued to work in partnership with ETSC. Discussions ensued with a plan to create a formal program leading to a baccalaureate in the science of nursing (BSN) for nursing students. By 1954, a BSN program had been developed, approved, and established at ETSC. The training school for nurses at Memorial (previously Appalachian Hospital) was slowly phased out in support of the ETSC program. Students who had completed their diploma program at Memorial Hospital were able to matriculate to ETSC as diploma nurses. In addition, they had already attended classes at the university, so much of the coursework had already been completed. Barbara Lewis graduated with a diploma in nursing from the Memorial (Appalachian) Hospital School of Nursing in 1954 and was the first student from Memorial Hospital to enroll in the newly approved ETSC science of nursing degree program. Because Lewis had taken the previous college courses at ETSC and had a diploma in nursing, it took her only one year to complete the additional ETSC nursing courses to meet the requirements for a BSN degree at ETSC. Lewis was the first nurse to graduate from ETSC's School of Nursing in 1955 with a BSN degree. This particular ETSC matriculation plan for students with a diploma in nursing could be viewed as the first RN-BSN nursing program in the state of Tennessee. Although Memorial Hospital remained open, the hospital's school of nursing permanently closed (Swartz, n.d.).

Founding of the American Nurses Association: A Focus on the Professionalism of Nurses

Nurse leader concerns about legal standards and professionalism were also foundational in the practice of nursing and central to the development of what is now called the American Nurses Association. Despite the establishment of formal Nightingale-based nursing principles in training schools for nurses across the United States, appropriate legal and educational standards were still lacking. It wasn't until 1893 that nurse leaders formally gathered at the World's Fair in Chicago for the first nurses' meeting in the United States to address both educational and professional concerns. In addition to nursing education, the professional practice of nurses and lack of regulations for nurses' training school graduates was discussed as a significant issue. Nurse leaders felt that the public needed to be protected from nurses who were poorly prepared for practice by ensuring that the graduate nurse was able to demonstrate competence through standards that were set by the profession.

In 1896, nurse leaders met in New York to discuss organizing a professional association for nurses, and by 1897 a meeting was convened at which the Nurses' Associated Alumnae of the United States and Canada was created. The purpose of this new organization was to establish a code of ethics; promote honor, financial interests, and usefulness of the nursing profession; and elevate the standard of nursing education (Flanagan, 1976). During that meeting the organization's constitution and bylaws were adopted, and Isabel Hampton was elected president. Hampton was considered a visionary in promoting the organization and growth of nursing. She was a strong advocate for the professionalism of nursing and also increasing the training time of nurses from two to three years. Another issue that plagued nurse leaders was the significant number of practitioners who were called "nurse" even though they had not received any formal nurses' training. Further, there was no certification method to indicate that a nurse was competent to practice. Hampton and the other nurse leaders agreed that in order for nursing to be recognized as a profession, there was a need for each state to establish, approve, and maintain a process of certification for graduate nurses. Thus, state nursing associations had to be organized in order to develop legislation to address these educational and professional issues. In 1899, Sophia Palmer, RN, one of the original founders of the American Society of Superintendents of Training Schools and a vocal advocate, led a movement to regulate the training of nurses through state registration (Bullough, Church & Stein, 1988). The goal of registering nurses required state legislation, a method of certification and the establishment of a nursing association in each state. In 1900, Hampton made the point that until registration could be enacted, nursing could not attain "its full dignity as a recognized profession" (Flanagan, 1976, p. 43).

State associations began to organize throughout the nation with a focus on promoting legislation to standardize nurses' training and regulate nursing practice. New York was the first state to organize in 1901 with the establishment of the New York State Nurses Association. Virginia, North Carolina, New Jersey, Illinois, and other states soon followed New York in establishing state nurses' associations. This effort ultimately resulted in legislation that included standards in nursing practice with a state law to control nursing practice and a process that would result in the registration of nurses through licensure after they had completed an approved training program within each state. This process would thereby separate trained nurses from those who were untrained. Each state would create a board of nursing, and in order to be licensed as a registered nurse, the applicant was required to have completed a formal training program. In addition, the graduate nurse was required to pass an examination that demonstrated competence in nursing. In 1902, Annie Damer, member of the first state Board of Nurse Examiners of New York, continued the call for registration, making a bold statement about the importance of professionalism in nursing

II. Evolution of Nursing Education/Professional Nursing

practice: "Nurses should demand recognition as a profession through granting of a proper certificate by a state constituted and maintained board of nurse examiners" (Flanagan, 1976, p. 44).

North Carolina became the first state to pass the Nurse Practice Act on March 3, 1903, followed by New Jersey (April 7), New York (April 24), and Virginia (May 14). In addition to North Carolina and Virginia, West Virginia (1907), Georgia (1907), Tennessee (1911), and Kentucky (1914; failed to pass in 1908) were the other states in Southern Appalachia that followed with enactment of state nurse licensure laws. The Nurses' Associated Alumnae was later renamed the American Nurses Association in 1911, and it had chapters established in each state (Flanagan, 1976; Shannon, 1975).

III

Early Nursing Practice

The Nexus of Medicine, Hospitals, and Nursing

Nursing practice in the core of Appalachia was reflective of the sociocultural, political, and demographic issues in the region during the late nineteenth to mid-twentieth centuries. Many nurses who were born and raised in the region during the late eighteenth and early nineteenth centuries had to attend training schools close to home and frequently remained in the region to practice. While some may have traveled a significant distance for their education, nurses from large cities outside of Appalachia, including New York City, Baltimore, Philadelphia, and Boston (and, in some cases, countries outside the United States), came to Appalachia to practice.

When considering the evolution of nursing education, professionalism, and practice, nurses' training schools, hospitals, and medicine cannot be viewed in isolation since they were closely interconnected with the healthcare of communities across the nation, including communities in the core of Appalachia. During the late nineteenth to mid-twentieth centuries, student nurses across the nation were not only germane to the hospital and work of the physician but also integral to the day-to-day operation of the hospitals, especially from an economic perspective. In addition to the required patient care, nursing students provided a vital service in supplying hospitals with convenient and inexpensive labor, which was part of their training school requirements.

Throughout this same period, most of the hospitals and medical schools that had been established in the Southern Appalachian region were located in larger, more populated cities. Until the late nineteenth century, hospitals in the core of Appalachia were few and far in between.

III. Early Nursing Practice

By the dawn of the twentieth century, hospitals gradually began to emerge within the Appalachian core, but they were established in the larger, more urban settings of the core region, leaving communities in the rural and isolated areas without access to a hospital or a physician. This lack created a need for nurses to provide healthcare to residents in the more isolated, rural areas, where frequently the nurses were the sole providers of healthcare for the entire community.

Tennessee Medical College (TMC), Lincoln Memorial University (LMU) and Affiliations in the Northeast

Knoxville, Tennessee, was fast becoming a major "hub" of healthcare during the late nineteenth and early twentieth centuries. While medical schools had been established in Memphis and Nashville during the early to mid–1800s, there were no formally organized medical schools in the east Tennessee region. During the mid–1800s, several attempts had been made to establish a medical school in Knoxville, but those attempts were unsuccessful. With the closest medical school located in Nashville, the distance created a hardship for individuals in the region who aspired to become physicians. In 1885, the idea of a medical school in east Tennessee surfaced again, and by 1889 ten physicians had met, formed a corporation, and established the Tennessee Medical College (TMC). The college opened that same year with 20 medical students. Reports suggest there was a nursing program; however, there is no evidence to indicate a formal nurses' training program ever existed (Platt & Ogden, 1969).

There were several small clinics and psychiatric facilities in Knoxville during the mid–1800s; however, the majority were short lived, and the city lacked an official hospital to care for its residents. Most of the healthcare in Knoxville took place in physician-run clinics or, in many cases, private homes where physicians, in addition to providing patient care, would often conduct surgeries on kitchen tables. Healthcare for the poor, however, was basically nonexistent. It wasn't until 1884 that the need for a city hospital for the poor resulted in the establishment of one of the first hospitals in Knoxville. The hospital was basic at best, so talks resumed about the need for a city hospital to adequately care for all of Knoxville's citizens, including the poor. These talks eventually led to the establishment in 1902 of the city-owned Knoxville General

Hospital, which also included a formal nurses' training program (Platt & Ogden, 1969).

At the same time, the medical faculty at TMC in Knoxville discussed the need for an academic partner in order to further the mission of their medical school. Financial issues had begun to plague the medical college, and overtures for financial assistance were made to Maryville College in Knoxville and Lincoln Memorial University (LMU) in Harrogate, Tennessee. The financial assistance for TMC included an academic link to a university, and LMU agreed to the union. In 1905, TMC became the Medical Department of Lincoln Memorial University (Hess, 2011).

It was determined that LMU/TMC needed a hospital site where medical students could practice with patients. Knoxville General Hospital could not accommodate the additional medical students, and early newspaper reports indicated LMU/TMC had difficulty locating a suitable site. The physician faculty at LMU/TMC finally decided to build a private hospital where the medical students would be able to practice. In 1906, Lincoln Memorial Hospital was built directly across the street from Knoxville General Hospital. Since nursing students staffed and provided patient care in hospitals, a training program for nurses was needed for the new LMU hospital, and by 1907 LMU had established a three-year formal nurses' training school. LMU boasted a couple of firsts in Tennessee nursing programs: LMU graduate Ophelia Hornsby was appointed in 1911 to Tennessee's first state Board of Nurse Examiners. LMU was also the first nurses' training program to include a male student. In 1913, John Brockman, graduate of LMU, became the first male registered nurse in east Tennessee.

For several years, the two hospitals and separate nurses' training programs operated simultaneously across the street from one another. Unfortunately, the legacy of TMC's financial and other associated problems continued to plague the renamed Medical Department of Lincoln Memorial University. In Flexner's 1910 report on "Medical Education in the United States and Canada," the results, for the most part, while not unlike other medical schools in the United States, were not complimentary toward the combined LMU/TMC institution. According to the report, the school adjoined a "neat," recently constructed hospital that appeared to be a private hospital of the faculty that student fees helped pay for. Weekly clinics often were not held, and there were no free wards. While the medical school building was considered "attractive"

III. Early Nursing Practice

on the outside, it was dirty inside, with continuing financial problems (Flexner, 1910; Hamer, 1930). LMU finally closed the medical school in 1914, and the students were transferred to the University of Tennessee Health Sciences Center in Memphis so they could complete their medical education. The LMU hospital continued to operate but at a loss, and by 1917 it was sold to Knoxville General Hospital. The LMU training school for nurses was then absorbed into Knoxville General Hospital's own training school.

The Connection Between Knoxville, Bellevue Hospital, and the Northeast United States

The medical and nursing profession in Knoxville had an early and sustained connection to Bellevue Hospital in New York City that began during the late nineteenth century. This connection appears to have emerged through medicine and Lincoln Memorial University. In 1897, Lincoln Memorial University was established in Harrogate, Tennessee, as a result of the fundraising efforts of Oliver Otis Howard, a resident of Maine and friend of Abraham Lincoln. As noted previously, LMU later became a partner with Tennessee Medical College in Knoxville when TMC's administration expressed a need for financial assistance and the university agreed to step in with funds (Hess, 2011).

Evidence of the affiliation between Knoxville medicine and Bellevue Hospital can be further observed in an early (circa 1915–1918) photograph depicting a Knoxville physician, Dr. H.K. Cunningham, standing next to a nurse seated at a desk in a hospital ward at Bellevue Hospital in New York City. In addition, Bellevue Hospital artifacts, including a Bellevue surgeon's cap referred to as a "kepi," were discovered in the medical history collection of the McClung Medical Museum in Knoxville.

In addition to the medical connection between Knoxville, Bellevue Hospital, and other hospitals in the Northeast, connections with the eastern part of the United States that most likely had a significant impact on nursing education and professionalism in the core of Appalachia had begun to emerge by the early twentieth century. There was a circuitous but integral connection between Knoxville General Hospital School of Nursing and nurse leaders Agnes Brennan, Jeanette Paulus, Lillian White, and Mary Littlefield. Jeanette Paulus (Pennsylvania born

Appalachian Nursing

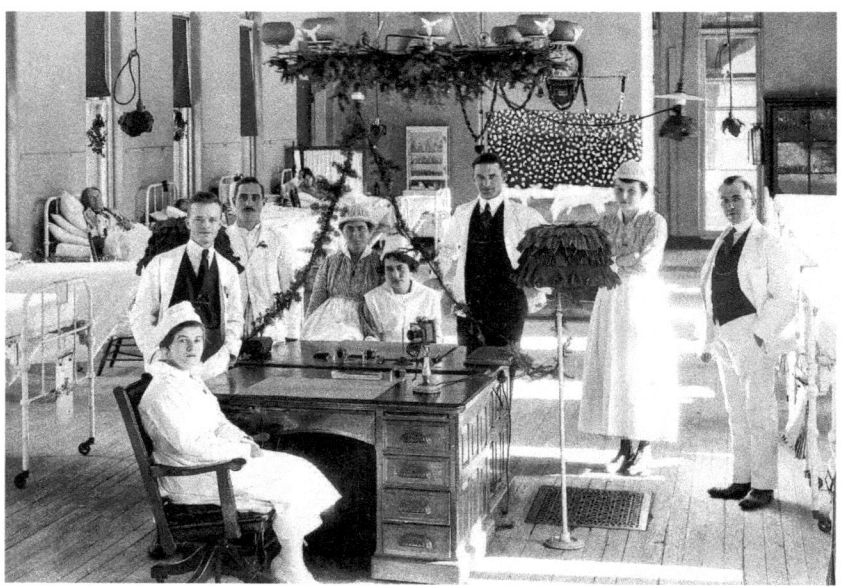

Dr. H.K. Cunningham from Knoxville, Tennessee, in Bellevue Hospital ward, New York City (leaning behind the nurse seated at the desk), c. 1916 (Museum at Mountain Home—ETSU College of Medicine, Johnson City, Tennessee, donated from the McClung Medical Collection).

and educated) was hired in 1902 as the first superintendent of Knoxville General Hospital's training school for nurses. Paulus was indirectly connected to Agnes Brennan and the nursing education program at Bellevue Hospital. Brennan, a nurse from New York, was an 1882 graduate of Bellevue Hospital's Training School for Nurses. She became the third superintendent of Bellevue's training school in 1888 and served in that role until 1902. Brennan was also a prominent member of the American Society of the Superintendents of Training Schools for Nurses and a strong advocate for excellence in the training of nurses. She wrote the paper "Comparative Value of Theory and Practice in Training Nurses," which was shared at the society's second annual convention in 1895. In her paper, Brennan suggested that practice in a nurses' training program was an essential component to nursing education. According to Brennan, "Practice helps to impress and retain in the memory the knowledge obtained by theory otherwise forgotten without the practical application" (Brennan, 1985, p. 65). It was reported that Brennan

III. Early Nursing Practice

knew every student at Bellevue and guided their training, and, under her direction, Bellevue Hospital's Training School for Nurses "prospered" (Bellevue Hospital Training School for Nurses, 1923).

Prior to her appointment at Knoxville General Hospital's training school for nurses, Jeanette Paulus graduated in 1891 from the Protestant Episcopal Hospital Training School for Nurses in Philadelphia and acquired eleven years of nursing experience in a number of reportedly "leading hospitals" in the East ("For Suffering Humanity," 1891, p. 5; "Jeannette Paulus," 1947, p. 1). The same year she was hired, Lillian White, another East Coast nurse, who was a 1902 graduate of the Protestant Episcopal Hospital Training School for Nurses in Philadelphia (the same nurses' training school as Paulus), was hired to serve as the director of nurses at Knoxville General Hospital. Together, both Paulus and White brought the Agnes Brennan/Bellevue/Protestant Episcopal Hospital influence to the Knoxville General Hospital School of Nursing. While at the Protestant Episcopal Hospital training school in Philadelphia, White trained under nursing superintendent Mary Littlefield. Littlefield was from New York and had graduated from Bellevue Hospital's Training School for Nurses in 1889. While a student at Bellevue, Littlefield trained under Brennan. Both Littlefield and Brennan became advocates for improvement in nursing education and were prominent members of the American Society of Superintendents of Training Schools for Nurses, later named the National League for Nursing Education. Paulus remained at Knoxville General Hospital as superintendent of its training school until 1909. During her seven-year tenure, Paulus became actively involved as a member of the first Tennessee State Board of Nurse Examiners, where she helped facilitate a bill to register graduate nurses in Tennessee. The registration bill was passed by the Tennessee state legislature in 1911 ("Jeannette Paulus," 1947, p. 1).

A later reverse connection between Bellevue Hospital's Training School for Nurses and the Knoxville General Hospital School of Nursing was identified through Ruby Hoyle. Hoyle was born in Knoxville and received her initial nurses' training through the Oppenheimer Institute, a private physician-owned hospital in Knoxville. Reportedly, the Oppenheimer Institute was a doctor-run hospital with a nurses' training school in Knoxville that opened in 1905. The school, however, was never listed as meeting guidelines set by the NLNE, nor did it appear they ever attempted to achieve Tennessee State Board of Nurse Examiners' approval. Hoyle went on to Bellevue Hospital's Training School

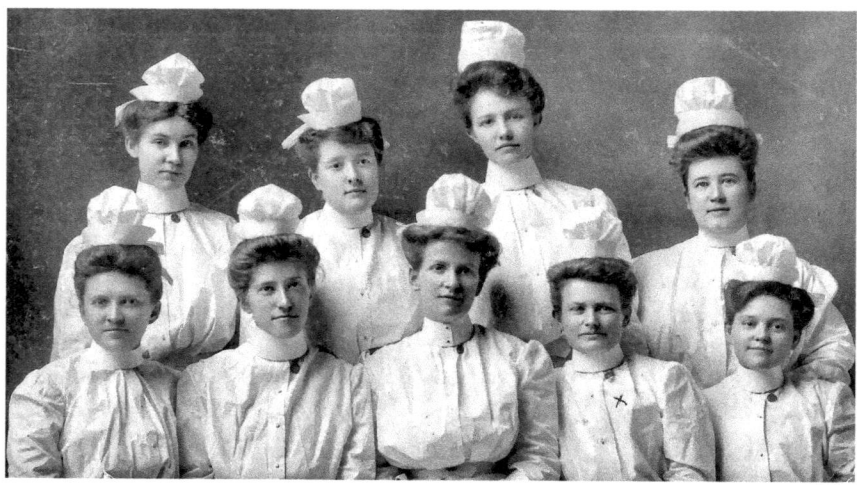

Knoxville General Hospital School of Nursing, first graduating class of 1905. Front row, from left: Ada Lawhorn, Mary Trigg Jackson, Lillian White (director), Ester Dodson, Parley Leinart; second row, from left: Maud Holloway, Lois Durkee, Emma Snowden, Sophie Cowan (courtesy Billie R. McNamara and the Knoxville General Hospital School of Nursing Alumni Society).

for Nurses and, returning to Tennessee after graduating from Bellevue, applied for registration from the Tennessee State Board of Nurse Examiners. On her 1920 application for registration, Hoyle indicated that she had completed further nurses' training courses in 1919 from Bellevue Hospital in New York City (Platt & Ogden, 1969; Tennessee State Board of Nurse Examiners, 1919).

Hospitals

Although small medical clinics and physician-run hospitals had been established in some smaller rural Southern Appalachian communities, their services were limited. Hospitals that provided full medical and surgical services were typically located in the larger urban centers of the region. Two known hubs of healthcare in the southeast core of Appalachia emerged in Tennessee and Virginia: Knoxville, Tennessee, and Roanoke, Virginia. While not considered large cities that were analogous to New York or Philadelphia, these towns were populated urban

III. Early Nursing Practice

centers in the core of Appalachia and central for healthcare and nursing education during the late nineteenth and early twentieth centuries.

Knoxville was one of the larger, more urban towns in east Tennessee that offered a number of hospitals and nurses' training schools within its environs as well as in the surrounding communities. Students from states outside the region traveled to Knoxville to attend the nursing programs at Knoxville General Hospital, Baroness Erlanger Hospital in Chattanooga, and later Fort Sanders Hospital in Knoxville. Some graduates stayed to practice in the Knoxville hospitals, but many returned to their hometowns or went on to practice in other areas of the Appalachian core and beyond.

Roanoke, Virginia (sometimes referred to as the "gateway to Appalachia"), was another hub of healthcare during the late nineteenth to mid-twentieth centuries. Roanoke boasted several well-equipped hospitals, nurses' training schools, and doctors and nurses that served as a central point for healthcare in the region. When smaller hospitals in the outlying communities in southwest Virginia could not adequately care for a patient, the patient was usually transferred to a larger hospital in Roanoke.

Role of the Staff Nurse

During the late nineteenth to mid-twentieth centuries, duties for hospital-based nurses (with the exception of the hospital superintendent or nurse anesthetists) were the same, whether the hospital was in New York City or a small rural community in Southern Appalachia. While the illness or injuries of patients may have varied due to regional or environmental differences, there was little difference in the nurse's responsibilities. The staff nurse provided care for the patients but also prepared and served food, maintained the environment of the hospital, took care of the hospital laundry, and performed housekeeping duties in the hospital. Nursing education programs provided training to address those responsibilities, but nurse leaders continued to voice their concerns that the hospital environmental needs frequently overshadowed the educational needs of the students in their training.

Role of the Hospital Superintendent

The superintendent of a hospital and training school had responsibilities that differed from those of the staff nurse, and those responsibilities could sometimes be overwhelming. While the superintendent was responsible for the hospital and overall patient care, she was also in charge of the hospital nurses, the training school, and the nursing students, in addition to occasionally providing direct patient care.

Amelia Young, born in 1890 in Crab Orchard, Tennessee, attended Lincoln Memorial Hospital Training School for Nurses in Knoxville. Following her graduation in 1911, Young worked in private-duty nursing for a few months until she was approached by a group of doctors who had just established Memorial Hospital, a small physician-owned hospital in Johnson City, Tennessee. They offered Young the position of hospital superintendent and chief nurse. Her position was described in a letter dated April 17, 1911, from Dr. Matthews, president of the new hospital:

> What we shall require of a superintendent is to take full charge of the house and its belongings and manage its affairs; to have charge of the nurses and help with their training, and to help nurse and care for the patients; all these duties to be performed in accordance with and by the advice, help and direction and orders of the Board of Directors. We realize this could be a rather large undertaking for one person, but we are men of sense and reason and shall not require more that it is possible for one person to perform [Stahl, 1989, p. 21].

Young accepted the position for $50 per month with room, board, and laundry; she was required to be available twenty-four hours a day. The hospital had ten beds, a small operating room, a kitchen, and a dining area. Young was provided with two student assistants, one with two years of training and the other a new student probationer without training. In her memoirs, Young recalled an especially stressful day when she was preparing the operating room for one of the doctors:

> My operating room had sterilizers heated by oil burners. One of my worst days was, when I was all ready for Dr. Miller and his assistant from Knoxville who were to do an appendectomy. I took his bag of instruments to sterilize, and found on opening the door that my sterilizer was pouring out black smoke and everything was covered with oily soot. I finally got things cleaned up and the operation went smoothly and the patient made a good recovery.

Six months later, Young resigned her position:

> I found this a lot of responsibility for a girl not yet twenty-one years of age, so in October of that year decided to accept an offer by Metropolitan Life

III. Early Nursing Practice

Insurance Company in Knoxville to start their visiting nurse program offered to their industrial policy holders.... This program, a new venture, got off to a good start and was used and appreciated [Harshman, 1982, p. 12].

GRACE MCBRIDE

Not unlike Amelia Young, Grace McBride also became disillusioned with her role as superintendent at the Highlands Sanitarium in Chattanooga, Tennessee. Born in 1885, McBride was raised in Ohio and, after attending one year of college, decided to pursue nursing. She enrolled in and graduated from a basic two-year nurses' training program at Philadelphia School for Nurses in Pennsylvania. McBride's original plan following graduation in 1908 was to return home to help care for her ailing father and practice as a private-duty nurse. However, her father died before her return home. McBride then decided to further her education in nursing. In 1909, she entered the nursing program at Bellevue Hospital in New York City, well known for its Nightingale-based principles in nursing education. According to her family, McBride was familiar with Bellevue's reputation for its nurses' education training program and had always wanted a Bellevue diploma. She completed her training program at Bellevue and graduated in 1911.

McBride subsequently moved to Chattanooga, Tennessee, to live with her sister. For a short time, she practiced private-duty nursing; however, it was not steady income. In 1912, McBride applied to Highlands Sanitarium, a hospital in Chattanooga that specialized in maternity cases and women's health. She accepted the offer of a full-time nursing position. Two months later, McBride was promoted to superintendent of nurses. Her duties as superintendent included general management of the hospital, ordering hospital supplies, paying bills, training nursing students, supervising the hospital nurses, housekeeping, laundry, and maintenance staff. In a letter to her family that year, McBride wrote:

> Since I came out here I have been through enough to write a book on.... Am sorry not to be with you now, but am so busy I can hardly think of home. Everything has been turned over to me and if it does not go, I do not think it will be because I am not rushing things, because it is quite a matter of concern to some of these people. In the morning we operate. There will be at least four operations this week, so we expect to be quite busy.... I am ... not over worked but would rather have a harder place and get $50.00 a month where one can have some satisfaction in their work, than to be at place like this at $70.00 a month.... I know that one can never find a place where

things go just to suit a person, but I surely have been turned against this.... I am going to stick to it if I can for a while [McBride, 1912, pp. 1–2].

McBride remained as superintendent at Highlands Sanitarium until 1914, when she made the decision to become a missionary and left Chattanooga to attend the Southern Baptist Convention Woman's Missionary Union Training School in Louisville, Kentucky. Miss A.E. Grass replaced McBride as superintendent and head nurse at Highlands Sanitarium.

Vesta Swartz

Toward the middle of the twentieth century, as the profession of nursing and nursing education matured, nursing superintendents gained more autonomy in their role. In 1941, Vesta Swartz, a graduate of the University of Maryland Hospital School of Nursing in Baltimore, was appointed superintendent of Appalachian Hospital's School of Nursing in Johnson City, Tennessee. Swartz was a visionary and took a progressive approach to nursing education by implementing a recommendation from the 1923 Goldmark Report to integrate hospital-based nurses' training with university-based academic coursework (Committee for the Study of Nursing Education, 1923). As noted earlier, Swartz became the architect of a partnership between the Appalachian Hospital and East Tennessee State College (ETSC). She worked with the administration at ETSC, and by 1943 Appalachian Hospital and ETSC had reached an agreement in which Appalachian Hospital nursing students would take college courses for credit during their training at the hospital. By 1949, ETSC and Appalachian Hospital established a formal affiliation. Per the agreement, nursing students received their first nine months of coursework (including physiology, psychology, sociology, principles of nursing, English, microbiology, chemistry, nutrition, and cooking) at ETSC. The students' clinical training remained at Appalachian Hospital. This university/hospital affiliation ultimately led to the establishment of the baccalaureate in the science of nursing (BSN) program at ETSC in 1954 (Swartz, n.d.).

Nurse Anesthetists

In addition to the nursing superintendent and staff nurse, another hospital-based role was that of the nurse anesthetist.

III. Early Nursing Practice

Dating back to the nineteenth century, nurses would frequently administer anesthesia to patients undergoing surgery; however, it wasn't until 1877 that Sister Mary Bernard became the first nurse to specialize in anesthesiology (Bankert, 1989). With the exception of St. John's Hospital in Illinois in 1879, where the surgeons trained nurses in the administration of chloroform, there were no formal training programs for nurses until 1889, when Dr. William Mayo established a nurse anesthesia training program at St. Mary's Hospital in Rochester, Minnesota (Ray & Desai, 2016). Since no formal nurse anesthetist training programs existed in Appalachia prior to the twentieth century, surgeons at hospitals instructed the nurses in how to administer anesthesia; the nurse would sit at the patient's head, administering the anesthetic through a cone-like piece of equipment. During the mid–twentieth century, however, there were nurses in the core of Appalachia who sought education to become specialized nurse anesthetists (American Association of Nurse Anesthetists, n.d.).

In east Tennessee, Archie Hobson, a 1919 graduate of Knoxville General Hospital and later supervisor of operations at the hospital, left

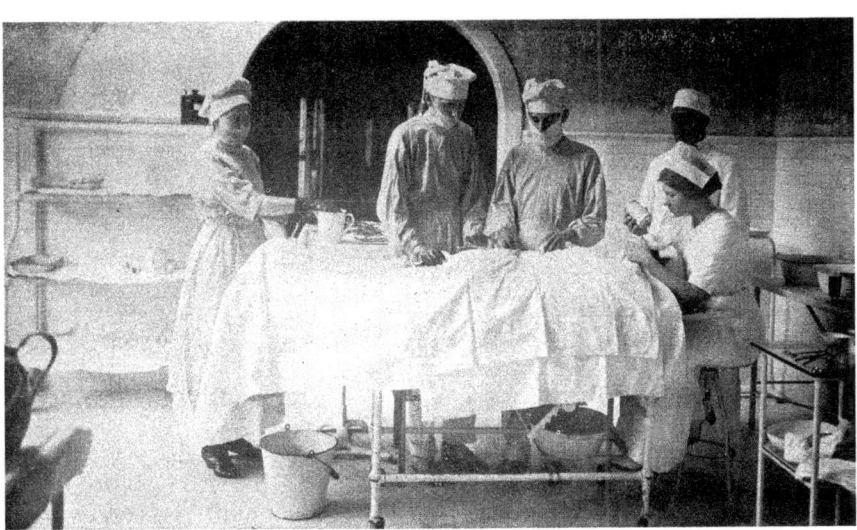

Doctors and nurses in the operating room at Miners' Hospital #1 in McDowell County, West Virginia, with a nurse administering the anesthesia, 1912 (West Virginia and Regional History Center, West Virginia University Libraries).

Knoxville around 1928 to enter the St. Mary's Hospital nurses' training program in anesthesia in Rochester, Minnesota. After completing the specialized training, she was well educated in ethylene administration; she then returned to Knoxville, where she practiced as a nurse anesthetist at St. Mary's Hospital and later at Fort Sanders Hospital. Hobson married Dr. Olin Rogers, chief of anesthetics at Knoxville General Hospital.

In addition to Hobson, there were other trained nurse anesthetists from the Knoxville area: Lula Mae Huhn received her nursing education at Vicksburg University, Charity Hospital, New Orleans, and in 1936 she practiced as a nurse anesthetist at St. Mary's Hospital in Knoxville. Zella Massengill graduated from the Knoxville General Hospital School of Nursing in 1926. She practiced for a short time at Knoxville General Hospital and later that year accepted a position at Jenkins Hospital in Kentucky; after a year, she returned to Tennessee. By 1933, Massengill was the superintendent of nurses at Howard Henderson Hospital in Knoxville. It is unknown when and where Massengill received her training in nursing anesthesia, but she was listed with Huhn and Hobson as three nurse anesthetists from Knoxville.

Charlotte Kyker was another nurse from the Knoxville area who later specialized as an anesthetist. She graduated in 1934 from St. Mary's Hospital School of Nursing in Knoxville, received her training in nursing anesthesia from Charity Hospital in New Orleans, and practiced as a nurse anesthetist at Holston Valley Community Hospital in Kingsport, Tennessee, and Sevier County Hospital in Sevierville, Tennessee ("Discovery of Ether," 1936; "New Face," 1936).

Psychiatric Hospitals

Psychiatric hospitals were another area of practice for nurses, although many well-known psychiatric hospitals were located in the larger urban areas outside the Appalachian core. While most general hospitals employed nurses as their superintendent, the role of superintendent in the psychiatric hospital was frequently filled by a physician. There were several psychiatric hospitals in the core of Appalachia, but the availability of information on nursing education in psychiatric hospitals is limited:

- Highland Hospital, Asheville, North Carolina
- State Hospital for the Insane (Broughton), Morganton, North Carolina

III. Early Nursing Practice

- East Tennessee Hospital for the Insane, Knoxville, Tennessee
- Southwestern Virginia Mental Health Institute (originally called the Southwestern Lunatic Asylum), Marion, Virginia
- Lakin State Hospital for the Colored Insane, Lakin, West Virginia
- Trans-Allegheny Lunatic Asylum, Weston, West Virginia

Prior to 1900, there was only one known psychiatric hospital with a formal nurses' training school in the core of Appalachia: the State Hospital for the Insane in Morganton, North Carolina (originally called the Western North Carolina Insane Asylum; later named Broughton Hospital in 1952). The Western North Carolina Insane Asylum was established by the state of North Carolina in 1883, when the Dorothea Dix Hospital in Raleigh could no longer accommodate the growing number of psychiatric patients in that region (Streeter, 2012). The name was changed to the State Hospital for the Insane in 1890. In the 1894 annual meeting of the American Medico-Psychological Association, psychiatric hospital superintendents discussed the need for nurses who were trained to intelligently care for the insane (Mitchell, 1894). Dr. Patrick Murphy, superintendent of North Carolina's State Hospital for the Insane, fully agreed that such a need existed and decided to establish a training school for nurses. He requested and was granted funds from the state of North Carolina to establish the new program, and by November 1895 the first psychiatric hospital training school for nurses in North Carolina was founded (Getz, 2009; Mitchell, 1894). Murphy believed that properly trained nurses would provide patients with kindness, structure, and discipline (Streeter 2011, 2012).

The school's training program was organized with clinical experience and lectures. Murphy and the hospital board envisioned their trained nurses would be able to practice in other psychiatric facilities and also provide private nursing care in the homes of patients who suffered not only from mental illness but also from physical illnesses. Murphy used the approach of moral therapy as a foundation for treatment of the mentally ill. This type of therapy was based on a humanitarian approach incorporating exercise and a non-stressful routine of work within a nurturing environment. The focus of treatment was on the mind, emotions, and soul as a way to reduce the psychological causes of mental illness (Getz, 2009). Central to nursing, moral therapy patients were treated with kindness and discipline while providing the patient

Appalachian Nursing

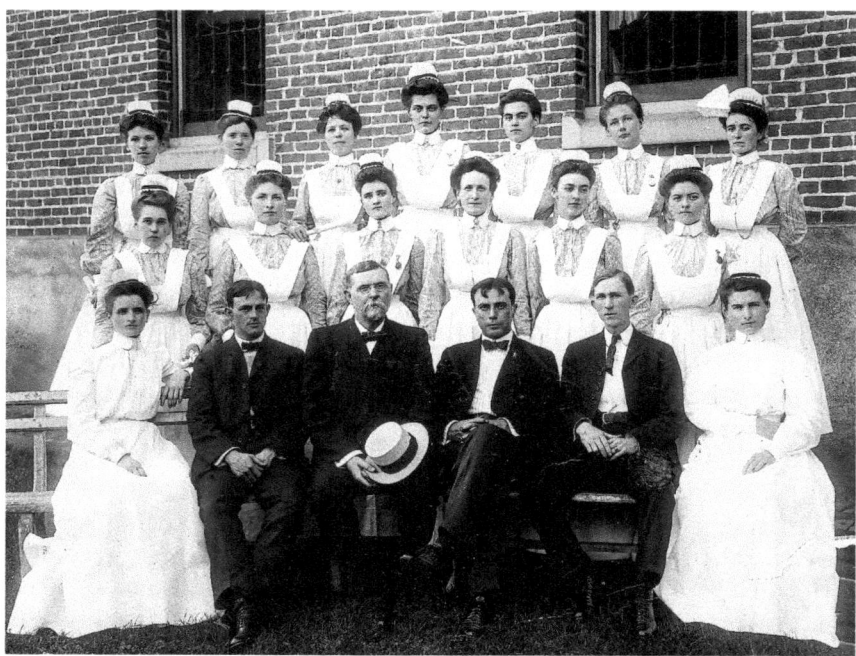

State Hospital for the Insane (Broughton Hospital), Morganton, North Carolina, nurses' training class (nurses, nursing students, and graduates), with Dr. Murphy, superintendent (first row, third from left), 1905 (Patrick Livingston Murphy Papers, #535, Southern Historical Collection, Wilson Library, University of North Carolina at Chapel Hill).

with a structured environment, daily routine, and meaningful activities (Streeter, 2011). The hospital had 712 beds and included laundry facilities, a farm, a garden, dining rooms, a chapel, and nurses' quarters. In 1896, the hospital employed 18 nurses. Miss S.E. Pitts, a nurse and graduate of Massachusetts General Hospital, Boston, was the nursing superintendent (Hodson, 1898).

Between 1895 and 1900, fifty-six nursing students were admitted to the training school. There was a three-month probation period with an additional training period of two years (Broughton Hospital History, 2016; Hodson, 1898). Male students were paid $13.50 per month, female students $11 per month. In the first class of students, twelve graduated to become nurses (Hobson, 1898). The hospital nurses were on duty 15 hours per day, including Sundays, with one afternoon from 2:00 to 6:00

III. Early Nursing Practice

p.m. off and one evening off from 7:00 to 10:00 p.m. each week (Broughton Hospital History, 2016). Murphy referred to the nurses' training school as vital to the success of moral treatment. He reported that his patients were better cared for and received more attention from the nurses as a result of the training, and there were fewer complaints of harsh treatment. He attributed an improved patient recovery rate to the better care provided by the nurses. He also believed these patients who recovered and were discharged would have died had it not been for the nurses' care and attention (Getz, 2009; Murphy, 1897, p. 14). The training school for nurses operated until 1962 and later became a clinical site.

Southwestern Lunatic Asylum

Originally named Southwestern Lunatic Asylum in Marion, Virginia, this psychiatric hospital opened in 1887 with two patients from Washington County, Virginia. In 1902, the name was changed to the Southwestern State Hospital. The hospital was set up with an operating room, gardens, a bowling alley, horse and dairy barns, and a farmhouse. Patients grew vegetables, raised cattle and pigs, and received treatment that included a healthy diet with fresh vegetables and an emphasis on outdoor exercise. In 1905, Lena J. Sprague from New York was hired as the first registered nurse at the hospital. By 1910, there were 34 nurses employed by the hospital, most of them from Virginia (1910 census). Sprague left prior to 1913 when she accepted a supervisory position at the Government Hospital for the Insane in Ogdensburg, New York.

By the 1950s, care of the psychiatric hospitalized patient became focused on a comprehensive team approach that included psychiatric social workers and staff from other departments. In a 2013 oral history study with former attendants who had worked at the psychiatric hospital during the mid-twentieth century, respondents commented on how increased regulation and a focus on professionalism had impacted their duties. A significant aspect of this new policy was related to administering medications, in which the responsibility was turned over to professionally trained nurses. This new policy wasn't particularly embraced by some staff:

> Well, the nurses were different, We got in new ones who had all sorts of rules for everyone to follow. There was all sorts of things that we, the aides, couldn't do no more, like give out the meds. I remember when one nurse

who was younger than me told me that I couldn't go to the medicine cabinet no more. I told her that I had worked there for over twenty years and I had never once taken anything out of that medicine cabinet and I certainly wasn't going to now. ... It was just different having new people around you telling you that you couldn't do something that you had been doing for years [Schrift, Cavender, & Hoover, 2013, p. 104].

HIGHLAND HOSPITAL

Highland Hospital (originally named Dr. Carroll's Sanitarium) in Asheville, North Carolina, was established in 1904 by Dr. Robert S. Carroll; it was a 65-bed private patient mental institution catering to celebrities and society's privileged. In 1912, the name was changed to Highland Hospital.

Nurse theorist Hildegard Peplau from New York City had received her master of arts degree in teaching and supervising psychiatric nursing at Teachers College, Columbia University, in 1947. While visiting her brother for the holidays that year in Asheville, Peplau made the decision to move from New York City to North Carolina; she subsequently applied for and accepted a nursing position at Highland Hospital. In the beginning, Peplau worked on the hospital wards. Dr. B.T. Bennett, the medical director, was a strong advocate in education for nurses, and his goal was to establish a psychiatric postgraduate nursing program at the hospital. When he learned of Peplau's background, Bennett offered her the position of nursing education director for a postgraduate program in psychiatric nursing. Peplau accepted the offer and developed the nursing program (Bullough, Sentz, & Stein, 1992; Callaway, 2002).

In March 1948, a tragic fire at Highland Hospital took the lives of nine women, including Zelda Fitzgerald, widow of F. Scott Fitzgerald. It was found the fire had been deliberately started by the night nursing supervisor (a former patient), who later confessed to over-sedating the patients she did not like, locking the patients into their rooms, cutting the phone lines, and setting the fire. The hospital was sold to Dr. Charmen Carroll, who offered Peplau the directorship and a partnership in the hospital. However, the tragedy had taken a toll on Peplau. She declined the offer and moved back to New York City, accepting an academic position at Teachers College (Callaway, 2002).

III. Early Nursing Practice

Visiting/Rural Nursing, the American Red Cross, Public Health, and Metropolitan Life Insurance

The roots of professional visiting nursing in the United States can be traced to England in 1859, when the wife of William Rathbone, a philanthropist and friend of Florence Nightingale, died. Rathbone had hired a local nurse to tend to his wife during her illness and believed that the services of trained nurses should be expanded to providing nursing care in the homes of the sick poor. Rathbone's vision evolved from not only personal experience with his ill wife but also Nightingale's theory of hygiene combined with proper nurses' training and prevention of disease. Rathbone theorized that in addition to providing care, nurses could teach patients how to correct or prevent the underlying causes of disease (Nightingale, 1890).

Nightingale expanded on Rathbone's thoughts:

> The trained district nurse [under the doctor] nurses the child or bread-winner back to health without breaking up the home.... The nurse also teaches the family healthy and disease-preventing ways by showing them her own in practice in their home.... Here, in the family, she meets them on their own ground. Besides nursing the patient, she shows them in their own home how they can help in this nursing, how they can be clean and orderly [Nightingale, 1890, pp. x, xi, xiv, xv].

With Nightingale's suggestion of starting a training school for district (visiting) nursing, Rathbone established and funded a training school for district nursing in Liverpool in 1863. His idea for district nursing, with the support of Nightingale, had taken root in England and most likely was the genesis of professional visiting nursing in the United States, where nursing expanded beyond the hospital and into the home (Rathbone, 1890).

In 1877, a similar venture emerged in the United States through the Women's Branch of the New York City Mission when trained nurses were first sent into the homes of poor patients in New York City. Lillian Wald and Mary Brewster, both graduates of the New York Hospital School of Nursing, envisioned a visiting nurse service similar to what had been established in England, with nurses whose training was also based on Nightingale's influence along with principles of public health and education. Wald and Brewster operationalized their vision for professional visiting nursing in 1893, with the establishment of the Henry Street Settlement, where the role of a visiting nurse with a public health perspective emerged. The actual term "public health nurse" in the United States can be traced to the settlement as the Henry Street nurses began providing visiting nurse healthcare and public health services to the poor in New York City. Wald's foreword in Marguerite Wales' 1941 book *The Public Health Nurse in Action* read, "We Called Our Enterprise Public Health Nursing" (Wales, 1941, p. xi). The Henry Street Settlement soon became the model and genesis of the Public Health Nurse and Visiting Nurse Association of New York.

Wald understood that the visiting nurse had a close relationship with the neighborhood, where the nurse's services went beyond physical care to address the environmental, financial, and social issues impacting the patients and neighborhoods they served. In 1909, Wald established a collaboration between the Henry Street Settlement and the Metropolitan Life Insurance Company. Metropolitan Life was founded in 1863 by New York businessmen under the name National Union Life and Limb Insurance Company. In 1879, industrial insurance for workers and their families was added to the program. Through this program, health education and prevention were provided to the workers and families through pamphlets; however, it was determined that distributing pamphlets was not sufficient and that nurses could be sent to the homes of policy holders. Wald worked together with Metropolitan Life to create a service to provide visiting nurse services to policy holders' homes through the Henry Street Settlement. The Metropolitan agent would contact the settlement when a home visit to one of the policy holder families was needed. The Henry Street nurse then made a visit to the Metropolitan Life policy holder family, providing treatment and education in hygiene and illness prevention (Metropolitan Insurance Company, 1914). The Henry Street visiting nurse association was paid $.50 for the home visit.

Although at first this service was provided in New York City and other large eastern and Midwest cities, Metropolitan Life Insurance Company later decided to expand its visiting nurse services to the rural areas of the United States, including the core of Appalachia. In some areas, where Metropolitan Life had no organized service or office, they often collaborated with other agencies in order to provide needed services. In those areas where Metropolitan Life offices existed, they were also the funding agency for other public health services, and by 1909 they began to establish a visiting nurse service in the core of Appalachia.

III. Early Nursing Practice

In addition to the New York Henry Street connection, Metropolitan Life was listed in 1909 as having a visiting nurse organization in Henderson, Kentucky; Chattanooga and Knoxville, Tennessee; and Clarksburg, West Virginia (Hamilton, 1989; Waters, 1912).

Amelia Young (Cox), superintendent of nurses at Memorial Hospital in Johnson City, Tennessee, had heard that Metropolitan Life was starting a visiting nurse service in the region and establishing its first office in Knoxville. Young decided to resign her position at Memorial Hospital and, in 1912, was hired to start Metropolitan Life's visiting nurse program. She was paid on a per-call basis, similar to the Henry Street arrangement with Metropolitan Life. Many of Young's patients and families lived in what she referred to as "slum conditions." Young felt that the Metropolitan Life program was effective but was concerned that there was no program to care for patients with tuberculosis. She attended a women's club meeting, shared her concerns, and then took a couple of women with her on visits to her tubercular patients. Young gained the support of prominent women in the community, and, through newspaper publicity, interest grew to the point that the Beverly Hills Sanitarium for tuberculosis patients on Black Oak Ridge was established by the Knoxville Civitan Club (Harshman, 1982).

The health conditions in Knoxville were another issue Young encountered in her work with Metropolitan Life. In her memoirs, Young stated, "The health conditions were so bad in Knoxville, I sometimes felt like a sprinkler pot trying to put out a great big fire and sometimes felt overwhelmed with responsibility" (Harshman, 1982, p. 13). Young had married and was living in Maryville, Tennessee, a suburb of Knoxville, when she learned Metropolitan Life Insurance Company was starting yet another nursing service program, this time in Maryville. She applied for and was accepted as an on-call visiting maternity nurse. Young was on call for maternity cases and paid $1 for maternity visits in which a bath for both the mother and the baby was provided. For advisory visits, she received $.75 per visit. In addition, Young developed a service for private-duty maternity nursing in which she charged $2 per visit and $5 to assist the doctor during delivery. Young took several years off to raise a family and moved back to Crab Orchard, Tennessee, her childhood home on the Cumberland Plateau (Harshman, 1982).

In 1934, Young became involved with the Homesteads Project in Crab Orchard, a government-funded rural resettlement program developed during the Depression in which 200 homesteader families were given the opportunity to work in exchange for a home and farmland on the Cumberland Plateau in Cumberland County. Young became the project nurse for the homestead community, making home visits to the families, most of which were maternity cases. She commented, "Having done home nursing for the Metropolitan Life Insurance Company in Knoxville and Maryville, I was well qualified to do home nursing" (Harshman, 1982, p. 46). Over a period of five years, Young delivered 250 babies, including one delivery in a barn (Harshman, 1982).

The American Red Cross, Lillian Wald, and Public Health

The American Red Cross was organized under the national headquarters in Washington, D.C., with regional jurisdictions. While known for its role in nursing during wartime, the Red Cross also had a prominent presence in visiting nursing and public health, both in cities and in rural areas across the United States. The jurisdictions in the core of Appalachia were arranged according to geographic area: Virginia and West Virginia were organized under the auspices of the Eastern Area in Alexandria, Virginia; Kentucky, North Carolina, Tennessee, and Georgia were in the Southeastern Area, Atlanta, Georgia.

Well known for the establishment of the Henry Street Settlement, Lillian Wald was a high-ranking member of the American Red Cross in New York State. Wald valued the work of the Red Cross and fully understood the need to provide nursing services to rural communities and small towns across the United States that had been identified by the Red Cross. She echoed the need and believed that the American Red Cross would be the best organization to undertake and provide professional visiting nursing services with a public health approach that expanded beyond urban areas to the rural and remote regions throughout the nation. In 1910, Wald wrote a letter to Jacob Schiff, a prominent member of incorporators of the American Red Cross, asking for support in creating an American Red Cross public health nursing service. In her letter, Wald made an appeal that a rural nursing service should be national in scope, and, "in my opinion, it would be much more desirable for the Red Cross to take up this work than it would be to organize another national society" (Dock et al., 1922, p. 1214). Wald added that the headquarters should be in Washington, D.C., with a trained nurse who would be a traveling supervisor. She also suggested local

III. Early Nursing Practice

chapters across the country with nurse supervisors to oversee the service. Wald believed that such an organization would also inspire students in nurses' training schools to consider postgraduate training at Teachers College, where potential scholarships could possibly be provided by the organization.

Wald's letter was shared at the annual 1910 Red Cross meeting in Washington. The request was not immediately approved; however, the American Red Cross, aware of the need for nurses in rural areas of the United States, had been impressed by the work of Lydia Holman in a remote and isolated community in North Carolina. In 1911, Schiff agreed to establish a fund for the establishment of a Red Cross rural nursing service; a year later, he offered a $100,000 endowment in securities. In addition, Mrs. Whitelaw Reid (wife of an ambassador and philanthropist) promised an annuity of $1,000 that increased to $2,000, and the rural nursing project was approved.

After assurance of the generous contributions, the American Red Cross agreed to organize a rural nursing service for a one-year trial period in every state in the nation. Fannie Clement, RN, was appointed superintendent of rural nursing (Dock et al., 1922). Introduced in 1912, this new department of the American Red Cross was named the Rural Nursing Service, incorporating concepts of public health into nursing visits in rural areas of the United States. The nursing services included assisting communities to secure services for their needs, consulting, and supervising these services without acquiring local financial responsibility (Dock et al., 1922). The one-year trial was successful, and, in 1913, the title Rural Nursing Service was changed to the Town and Country Nursing Service, so that both rural and small urban towns would be included in the service. Because of its prominent role in rural nursing, the Red Cross determined that appropriate education in public health principles was essential for its rural nurses. By 1915, the Red Cross had developed a training program so there was standardization of the work and qualification of its public health nurses (Dock et al., 1922; Ehrenfeld, 1919). The aim was to provide education and access to resources by specially trained nurses who delivered care to the community, without the community having to assume financial responsibility, and it paved the way for local effort and funding while also providing the foundation for public health nursing under the auspices of each state. The Town and Country Nursing Service later transitioned to the title of Red Cross Public Health Nursing (Dock et al., 1922; Fox, 1932).

Appalachian Nursing

The focus of Red Cross Public Health Nursing was to provide Red Cross chapter activities in communities that lacked public health nursing services. The Red Cross used its funds to pay for those services until state or municipal funds could take over the costs (Ehrenfeld, 1919).

In 1912, the National Organization for Public Health Nursing had been established, with Lillian Wald elected as president, and Lydia Holman, in Altapass, North Carolina, as one of the directors of the organization. Its purpose was to develop nursing standards and a formal education program for public health nursing (Hubbard, 1950). The Red Cross continued to meet the public health needs of residents in the small, rural towns in the core of Appalachia as well as in other rural areas throughout the United States. By the 1920s, the Red Cross Bureau of Public Health became the Red Cross Public Health Nursing Service. Eventually the states began to recognize the work of public health nurses and needs of the residents in the region to the extent that the Shephard-Towner Act of 1921 provided funding for states to develop programs for promotion of education and services to address the needs of mothers and infants. In 1923, Public Health Nursing became a unit of the American Public Health Association.

Red Cross and the Delano Nursing Service

Another service specific to rural nursing was the Delano Red Cross Nursing Service established 1919 in honor of Jane Delano. Delano was director of nursing in the American Red Cross from 1909 until her death ten years later. In memory of her parents, Delano left $25,000 in her will to the American Red Cross to be used for the support of "one or more visiting nurses ... to be known as the Delano Red Cross Nurse, or Nurses." In addition, Delano granted the American Red Cross the rights and interest in royalties derived from books written or published by her. This would have included her *American Red Cross Textbook on Home Hygiene and Care of the Sick*, originally published in 1913. This volume covered everything from symptoms of disease to hygiene in the home, bed making, baths, babies, children, medicines, communicable diseases, and emergencies (Delano & Strong, 1918). By 1924, there were five Delano Red Cross nurses: Edith Spiers was appointed to Maine in September 1922; Margaret Harry, appointed to Macon County, North Carolina, October 1922; Stella Fuller, appointed to Alaska, October 1922; Emily Thornhill, appointed to Buchanan County, Virginia, January 1924; and

III. Early Nursing Practice

Janet Worden, appointed to Idaho, February 1924. The Delano nurse resided in isolated communities providing nursing care and teaching families about health. It was considered an honor to be selected as a Delano nurse since the requirements called for special qualifications that included perfect health and courage, along with personal characteristics of diplomacy, determination, and perseverance, as well as a nurse who would encounter hardships while embracing rural life. She also had to demonstrate leadership, as she would become central in the community (Carrying on for Jane A. Delano, 1937; Noyes, 1924).

Visiting Nurse Services in Southern Appalachia

The roots of visiting and public health nursing in Southern Appalachia were founded in the underlying tenets of Florence Nightingale, Lillian Wald's Henry Street Settlement, and the American Red Cross, where concepts of public health and social services were central in providing nursing care not only to residents in large cities but also to the rural and remote communities of the United States. In 1909, Yssabella Waters developed a directory of organized visiting nurse services that provided an overview of what trained visiting nurses were doing across the nation. Waters identified three organizations in the core of Appalachia that were the first known organized visiting nurse services in the region: Women's Christian Temperance Union Settlement, Hindman, Kentucky; Lydia Holman (individual), Altapass, North Carolina; Flower Mission and Associated Charities, Visiting Nurse Department, Asheville, North Carolina (Waters, 1909).

Hindman, Kentucky (a small, isolated community in the mountains of Kentucky, 45 miles from the nearest railroad)
Organization: Women's Christian Temperance Union Settlement

- One nurse, irregular hours
- Surgical, medical, obstetrical, contagious, tuberculosis
- Had a settlement house (log cabin) with 18 rooms (Hindman Settlement School) where teachers, students, and a visiting nurse resided
- Nurse provided lessons in home nursing and homemaking
- Large number of tuberculosis patients; plan made for a tuberculosis camp during summer with nurse demonstrations for prevention and cure of tuberculosis

Appalachian Nursing

Altapass, North Carolina (1902)
Organization: self—Lydia Holman

- One nurse, irregular hours
- Surgical, medical, obstetrical, contagious, tuberculosis
- Closest reliable physician located many miles from the community
- Large district; nurse rode her horse from visit to visit and carried supplies strapped to her saddle
- Distances between cases ranged from 5 to 20 miles; needs of patients sometimes exceeded that within traditional nursing care

Asheville, North Carolina (1908)
Organization: Flower Mission and Associated Charities, Visiting Nurse Department

- Two nurses (one a senior nursing student)
- Student conducted the general home visits and was supervised by the graduate nurse. Calls for service came from numerous sources. For patients without medical assistance, the case was reported to the Associated Charities physician.

While the American Red Cross and public health nursing had been established in larger U.S. cities during the 1890s, by the turn of the century these services began to make their way gradually to more rural areas across the United States, including the Southern Appalachian region. Inspired by the work of Lydia Holman, and supported by Lillian Wald, the American Red Cross led an effort to establish an organized approach to provide visiting nursing and public health services in the Southern Appalachian region. The Red Cross Rural Nursing Service was created expressly for the purpose of bringing nursing care to patients in rural communities where healthcare was limited or, in most cases, nonexistent. The core of Appalachia fell into that category, and the need was significant.

To be accepted into the Red Cross Rural Nursing Service, nurses were required to have had two years of training in a recognized nursing school and be of good character (Dock et al., 1922); to practice as a public health nurse, additional training in public health essentials was required. These courses were usually provided through Teachers College in New York and a number of colleges across the United States.

III. Early Nursing Practice

The Red Cross nurses not only provided nursing care in the home but also educated families in the community regarding hygiene and the prevention of disease. In addition, they would arrange for social and environmental services when necessary. Health education was central to the Red Cross nurse as a way to empower community residents in preventing illness and injuries. Red Cross nurses also offered in-person training classes to community residents on topics that included basic hygiene, first aid, and nutrition. In addition, the nurses provided the residents with books on healthcare, including hygiene, care of the sick, and other health-related topics (Delano & McIsaac, 1917).

By the early part of the twentieth century, the Red Cross, visiting/rural nursing, and public health had become the main areas of practice for nurses in the Appalachian region, which continued well into the mid-twentieth century. This approach to healthcare delivery was necessary in order to serve residents in the remote rural communities. In these areas, even small hospitals were a minimum of 20–50 miles away, requiring residents to cross mountains, rivers, and unpaved roads to reach a hospital. With limited access to hospitals and physicians, visiting nurses were the primary (if not the only) providers of medical care, and, in many cases, the nurse had to provide care that physicians would normally do (Plyler, 1980).

Visiting nursing, the American Red Cross, public health, and, to a certain degree, Metropolitan Life Insurance became interconnected in the region to the extent that services were provided to community residents through collaborative efforts, rather than in competition with one another. Working together, the Red Cross and public health nurses coordinated services between the rural communities that were without hospitals or adequate medical service and those in urban areas where hospitals and adequate medical services were available. This partnership was clearly evident during the 1950s when Wytheville, a small rural town in southwest Virginia, experienced a serious polio epidemic. Wytheville, which had limited resources, became overwhelmed when many residents in the community contracted polio. The community hospital and small doctor-run clinics in Wytheville were not prepared to care for polio patients. Not only was there a lack of proper equipment, but there were also few medical providers with expertise in polio treatment. The Red Cross and public health nurses stepped in and, together, worked with the doctors in Wytheville to transfer their polio victims to Roanoke Memorial Hospital, which was fully prepared with doctors, nurses, therapists, and equipment. One resident of Wytheville recalled, "Out in the country you could hear the sirens taking people to Roanoke who had polio. And we'd say Uh-oh, there's another case, because out in the country you could hear the sirens. It was spooky, it really was" (Jackson, 2005, p. 85). Another resident shared that the nurses at Roanoke Memorial Hospital "would pick up that little child and put it on their shoulder with no fear of contagion" (Jackson, 2005, p. 35).

Sadly, racial division was an issue during the polio epidemic in Wytheville. One person recalled an incident with an African American child who had contracted polio:

> We took her to Richmond. At that time, all the white children were going to Roanoke Memorial Hospital. They wouldn't accept her there. In the hot sun we sat in an ambulance up here on Main Street while Dr. Charlie Graham talked by phone with them in Roanoke, trying to make them admit her, but they would not. It took all that time to make the drive to Richmond, which we think may be what caused the paralysis in her jaw [Jackson, 2005, p. 40].

The polio epidemic in Wytheville also spawned an interest in the nursing profession. Jean Kitts Lester was a resident of Wytheville during the outbreak, and this event may have been the reason she became a nurse. Kitts Lester recalled:

> I am a nurse and I think the Polio epidemic had something to do with deciding to follow that dream. I went to Johnston Memorial Hospital that year. For my final paper, which was an essay, I chose to write on the polio epidemic of 1950. I got an A on it because my interviews were with real people! The other nurses had to use books and encyclopedias. My professor was excited that I got to talk with people that lived through it [Jackson, 2005, pp. 131–132].

Lillian White was a nurse who transitioned from an administrative role in nursing education to the American Red Cross. White was the second director of nurses at Knoxville General Hospital, serving from 1902 to 1907. She graduated from the Protestant Episcopal Hospital Training School for Nurses in Philadelphia in 1902 and, that same year, began her tenure as the nursing director at Knoxville General Hospital. White remained in that role for five years, and, for a number of years thereafter, she continued in an administrative role as superintendent of nurses at a number of nurses' training schools across the United States. She eventually became the assistant superintendent of nurses at the University of California in San Francisco. White was also a member of the National League of Nursing Education and had a strong interest in the professional education of nurses that was clearly evident when she wrote a 1909 journal article about the importance of the professional education of nurses.

As the American Red Cross began to mobilize for World War I in 1916, White decided to apply for enrollment in the Red Cross Nursing Service. On the application was a recommendation from the superintendent of Protestant Episcopal Hospital Training School for Nurses, where White had graduated, describing White as "a superior woman, capable nurse, unusual executor ability, takes kindly to responsibility" (U.S., American Red Cross Nurse Files, 1916–1959, n.d.). When on the application White was asked to indicate why she wished to become a Red Cross Nurse, she wrote:

> The care of the sick and wounded in time of war was the primary object in organizing the Red Cross, however no effort was made in this country to establish an adequate nursing service until after its reorganization in 1905 when several states enrolled nurses, gradually so extended in time of peace, the need of trained nurses became evident and in 1909, an affiliation was formed with the American Nurses' Association.... My reasons for desiring enrollment are for teaching and organization purposes [White, 1909; U.S., American Red Cross Nurse Files, 1916–1959, n.d.].

White was accepted into the American Red Cross in 1916 and became the director of nursing for the Pacific Division (Kernodle, 1949, p. 499). In 1922, she resigned from the Red Cross due to her mother's ill health and need for assistance. In response to White's resignation letter, Clara Noyes, national director of the Red Cross Nursing Service, signed White's Efficiency Record with the following notation: "Miss White was eminently satisfactory as a Division Director—interested, enthusiastic, and dearly loved by those with whom she worked" (U.S., American Red Cross Nurse Files, 1916–1959, n.d.).

Rural and Public Health Nursing Practice in the Core of Appalachia

Prior to the first formal appointment of a public health nurse with accorded official status in 1919, many nurses across the nation, including in the core of Appalachia, were practicing/visiting/public health nurse pioneers, who provided public health service without the formal designation. Such caregivers became an important and major source of healthcare for Appalachian residents, especially those in distant communities.

Appalachian Nursing

While some communities in the Appalachian core region may have had small hospitals or doctors' clinics, most healthcare resources were located in the larger urban settings in the region. Many residents, however, lived in remote and isolated, sometimes inaccessible areas, many miles from the railroad, where it could take hours by horseback (or sometimes on foot) to reach a doctor or the hospital. As a result, nurses went to the patients. This practice was commonplace throughout the region; if the patients could not come to the nurse, the nurse would visit the patients where they lived. White Rock Hospital in Laurel, Madison County, North Carolina, provided one example of how hospital nurses met the needs of the patient through home visits. Frequently, after the end of their shifts, nurses who worked at White Rock Hospital made visits on horseback to patients who sometimes lived twenty miles or more from the town and hospital. While a doctor resided in the hospital manse, it was often difficult for his patients to return to the hospital for follow-up care or monitoring once they were released. However, home visit services by one doctor and a few nurses were frequently limited due to the number of visits that were usually required to address their patients' needs. The doctor and his nurses sometimes made their visits together, or, in most cases, the nurses made the visits and kept the doctor informed of the patients' status.

As in many other communities across the core of Appalachia, the lack of professionally trained physicians and adequate medical care was a common problem due to the isolation of rural and remote communities throughout the region, in addition to the limited interest of physicians who preferred to practice in urban areas. The lack of available doctors in these remote communities created challenges that led to a different form of care provided by the nurses. In the absence of local doctors, visiting/public health nurses in the core of Appalachia became the sole source of healthcare, frequently supplying medical care for their patients that was normally performed by a physician. Such an approach notably differed from the traditional nursing care provided by nurses in large cities, such as New York or Boston. In an oral history interview, one public health nurse who had practiced in a remote area of North Carolina during the 1920s and 1930s described those differences. This nurse suggested the care provided by public health nurses in urban areas of the northern United States was very different from what was standard practice in the rural and remote regions of the South. One of the main differences was the shortage of professionally

III. Early Nursing Practice

trained physicians who could provide care to the communities in the isolated regions. This situation left the medical care that was normally covered by the doctors to be provided by the nurses instead. Another frequent challenge for nurses in the isolated communities was having to work with limited resources and supplies. These nurses had to rely on their own creativity, innovation, personal resources, and supplies. By contrast, in the larger cities and towns in the North, there usually was a sufficient supply of doctors to provide standard medical care to the patients, which, in turn, allowed the nurses to provide traditional nursing care for their patients, with adequate time to focus on their patients and psychosocial issues (Plyler, 1980).

By the turn of the century, nurses in the larger cities across the United States had become aware of the need for healthcare in the rural Southern Appalachian region. Those with a pioneer spirit answered the call. Many nurses, however, were not used to the differences between city living and the often-difficult living conditions in isolated areas that were far removed from the conveniences of a city. Some nurses, even those with a strong spirit of adventure, were not able to adapt to the inconveniences, remoteness of the region, or harsh travel conditions and decided to return home while others settled in, having grown fond of the community residents and their traditions, beliefs, values, and lifestyle. These pioneer nurses were determined to make a difference in the lives of those they served. They persevered despite the harsh conditions, bad weather, and inconveniences, eventually adapting to their environment. Originally considered outsiders, the pioneer nurses who stayed had found their life's work, dedicated themselves to helping people in this remote region of the United States, and ultimately became trusted and respected members of the community.

A Cross Section of Nurses Involved in Visiting Nursing and Public Health in the Core of Appalachia

Mary Trigg, Tennessee and Kentucky

In 1905, Mary Trigg was one of the first graduates from the Knoxville General Hospital School of Nursing in Knoxville, Tennessee. She originally wanted to be a doctor, but most medical schools at that time would not admit females, so Trigg decided to pursue nursing and, in 1902, enrolled in the first training class of eight nursing students at Knoxville General Hospital. While she was a student at Knoxville General, a tragic 1904 train wreck occurred in Jefferson County, Tennessee. Fifty-six people were killed and 106 injured. As Trigg recalled afterward,

> I had to operate the elevator at General to carry the injured to different floors. The hospital was small, Persons had to be put on mattresses in the halls, anywhere that space permitted. The wreck happened around 10AM. But it was late in the afternoon before Southern Railway train could bring the injured on flat cars to Knoxville. The train stopped at Bernard Ave. and the injured were carried on stretchers two blocks to the hospital [Prince, 1964, p. 49].

After graduation, Trigg practiced at both Knoxville General Hospital and Lincoln Memorial Hospital, where most of the patients were hospitalized as the result of railroad injuries. She was also a proponent of nursing registration and a member of a group of nurses that in 1911 went to Nashville to encourage the Tennessee State Legislature to establish a state board of nursing that would require nursing practice standards, oversight, and the registration of graduate nurses. The board was approved that same year, and Trigg became one of the first registered nurses in the state of Tennessee. In an interview, Trigg shared, "I would have been first, but they started registering Memphis and Nashville first" (Prince, 1964, p. 49).

Trigg also became active in the suffrage movement. In 1913, she and several other nurses from the area traveled by train to Washington, D.C., and marched down Pennsylvania Avenue fighting for women's rights. Trigg recalled how "the men up there nearly killed us … the police didn't give us any protection. We were mobbed several times and told to go home and have babies" (Prince, 1964, p. 49).

In 1914, Trigg transitioned from hospital nursing practice to serving as a visiting nurse in the coal country. She attended Teachers College in New York for the visiting nurse/public health training that was required by the Red Cross Town and Country Nursing Service and subsequently became supervisor for Red Cross nurses in Kentucky, where she taught the Red Cross course "Home Care of the Sick" (Lexington Herald, 1919). Trigg was a strong proponent of public health nursing and accepted a position as director of welfare for the mining camps at

III. Early Nursing Practice

Consolidated Coal Company in Letcher County, Kentucky. The mining company had a hospital in Jennings, Kentucky, staffed by a doctor with whom she worked. She visited other mining camps and took a medicine bag with her on those visits. Trigg covered several hundred miles per week and recalled riding mules and horses throughout the eastern Kentucky mountains in order to make her visits. In some places the paths were so steep that she would have to dismount and hold on to the horse's tail so that she could be pulled up the mountain. In 1922, Trigg returned to Knoxville, where she practiced for another seven years before retiring in 1929 (Prince, 1964).

Lydia Holman, North Carolina

Lydia Holman was one example of several prominent nurse pioneers who were born and educated outside Appalachia but made significant contributions in bringing healthcare to residents in remote and inaccessible areas in the Appalachian core region, where access to healthcare would otherwise have been nonexistent.

Holman's connection to North Carolina began in 1900 when she first came to Mitchell County, North Carolina. This was years before government funding became available for public health departments or services for the county. Holman was born in 1868 and received her nurse's training at Philadelphia General Hospital in Pennsylvania. While in Philadelphia, she was hired by a wealthy female patient with typhoid fever who needed nursing care at her vacation home in North Carolina. Holman accepted the position and soon arrived in Ledger, Mitchell County. In December 1900, she found the rugged mountainous community extremely isolated; residents were without many services, including a healthcare provider. Ledger was thirty miles from the closest railroad, with no paved roads, hospital, doctor, or trained nurses. Although Holman was considered a pioneer in rural North Carolina nursing, she was also an "outsider," having to earn the trust and respect of the community residents. At first the locals were suspicious and skeptical of the newcomer but soon became impressed with the care Holman provided for her patient and the patient's subsequent recovery. Gradually some residents began to seek Holman's services for their own illnesses and injuries. She was sometimes referred to as the "mountain doctor" or the "friendly nurse." In an article, Holman described the community and its residents:

Appalachian Nursing

> These mountain folk know nothing of trained nurses, anyone capable of looking after them in illness is, in their idea, a "doctor," so that from January to May, opportunities were many and varied, in visits made among their sick, to see their hopeless lack of intelligent care and their inability to get any treatment other than herb and root teas, poultices, or rubbings, given by the nearest friendly neighbor [Holman, 1907, p. 831].

Holman eventually began to fit into the community and enjoyed the rural lifestyle far removed from Philadelphia. However, after her first patient recovered, Holman found herself having to return to Philadelphia. However, she kept an eye on the prospect of returning to rural North Carolina and providing much-needed healthcare in this remote region. Holman also knew that she needed further practice outside of the hospital setting. To prepare herself, she spent two years gaining additional experience in maternal and child health by working with the poor in Philadelphia and later at the Henry Street Settlement, where she provided care to the poor and underserved immigrant community in New York City. While at the Henry Street Settlement, Holman began to receive letters from the residents of Ledger asking her to come back. She expressed concern about the people of Mitchell County, reminiscing afterward that "throughout the year there was with me an unhappy consciousness of the hardships and needs of the mountain folk I had left" (Holman, 1907, p. 832).

Holman later referred to their needs as of necessity, a sort of combination of country doctor and visiting nurse. By 1902, she returned to Ledger with an actual salary for specific duties that was paid by her former patient. There was an understanding that Holman would also provide healthcare to the mountain people who needed her services. Reaching the nearest hospital was difficult for residents in the remote areas of Mitchell County, as they would have to travel 30 miles over harsh terrain. Holman began making visits on horseback to those residents and, by December 1902, had established the Mountain Visiting Nurse Service, which was listed in the directory *Visiting Nursing in the United States* (Waters, 1912). As a recognized formal visiting nursing service in Altapass, Mitchell County, North Carolina, Holman's service was described as having irregular hours during which calls were answered when received. The service was listed as having one nurse (Lydia Holman), and the care included nursing services for medical, surgical, and obstetric cases. Most diseases were covered, including tuberculosis as well as other contagious diseases. Holman's services

III. Early Nursing Practice

also covered home visits. In cases when she was not able to make another visit for several days, Holman stayed with the patient to provide the family with instructions and demonstrations of proper care. Although most of Holman's visits fell within the province of acute illness and obstetrical cases, she sometimes would perform minor surgeries, addressing medical issues such as skin problems and tooth extractions. Dental issues were another significant problem in the region. Holman attributed these problems to the lack of an adequate toothbrush, describing the toothbrushes community residents used as being made from pieces of splintered wood dipped in snuff (Waters, 1912).

Holman had support from the Boston Committee, an organization that provided financial assistance for her work (this assistance included clothing, supplies, and other items for the residents of Mitchell County). Patients were charged for nursing care ranging from no fee to $10 based on distance and number of visits rather than the amount of time and work involved. In many cases, if the patients could not pay in cash, they would pay with what they had on hand, including chickens, produce from the farm, wood products, or whatever the patients had in generous supply.

The community residents embraced Holman's presence and the services she provided. One long-standing doctor in the community likewise approved of the work Holman had been doing and sent patients to her. However, there were several newer doctors who had recently come into the region and did not understand (or investigate) the circumstances under which Holman worked. These doctors took issue with Holman and her work with Mitchell County residents. They believed that Holman was exceeding her role as a nurse. Although these new doctors did not reside in, visit, or fully understand Mitchell County, the region, its health issues, and the lack of access to medical care, they decided to bring charges against Holman for practicing medicine without a medical license. According to Holman, they wanted to "get rid of her." The older country doctor in the community, however, did not feel threatened because he understood the region and fully supported Holman's work. In addition, Holman had the support of the county residents and administration. Eventually, the case against her was dismissed (Holman, 1918).

Holman delivered an annual informal report to the Boston Committee, in which she would provide a description of the work that she had done for the year. As an example in her report for 1917, Holman described the following service calls provided by her organization:

> 874 [f]or extracting teeth or have them treated. Infected sores, saw mill accidents, fractures, strains, foreign bodies in eyes, ears. Abscesses, carbuncles, infected glands.
> 22 pre-natal visits, furnishing layettes, distributing pamphlets.
> 682 visits to homes, acute chronic cases, living one-quarter to forty miles.
> 15 sent away for special examination, suspected cases pellagra, tuberculosis, rheumatism, appendicitis, gall stones, tonsils, adenoids, eyes.
> 17 house cases for minor ailments that required remaining over because they lived so far away.
> 19 "Flux" cholera morbus, all cared for in their homes; no losses. Diet and nursing.
> 21 visits to schools. Health talks. Loaned out at one time very sick-room article on the place, also sheets, pillowcases, towels from loan closet.

Holman went on to report that at least 1,600 calls had been made for a variety of needs that year. She believed that clothing supplied to the residents helped to prevent diseases such as "rheumatism, neuralgia, nephritis, and pneumonia," going on to say that supplying babies' layettes "helped prevent death, especially from 'boled' hives; babies no longer die of this where we work" (Holman, 1918, pp. 1–4).

Unpaved roads in Mitchell County went through the mountains; they were mostly impassable during the winter months and required Holman to make visits to her patients on horseback. She described the geography of the county in one of her reports: "This week we were called into one of the very remote places, where even a horse cannot travel without safety. We could travel ten miles on the train, then walk one and a half" (Holman, 1918, p. 7). Most residents lived in small log cabins with one or two rooms, open fireplaces, and sometimes windows. These mountain cabins were anywhere from five to twenty miles apart. Carrying her supplies strapped on her horse's saddle, Holman often rode 30 miles per day, taking care of a variety of conditions from tooth extractions to surgeries and obstetrics. During her visits, Holman provided the families she met with instructions and demonstrations. She referred to her work as follows:

> Often I ride from five to twenty-two miles to make a single visit.... I was in the saddle nearly all the time for three weeks and able to stop at home only long enough for baths and changes of clothing. The work is not always so hard and there are compensations—the blue sky, the everlasting hills, the

clear, exhilarating air, and the simplicity of the people. These all go to make my life here a happy one [Holman, 1907, p. 834].

She went on to describe one of her family cases:

> January 7...S. J. Apparently ivy poisoning, had been applying "cream and gunpowder," became infected, and came to have "risin" under arm opened, which I declined to do, but rubbed it with icthyol, using wet compresses of carbolic on the poison [Holman, 1907, p. 835].

With additional assistance from colleagues in Baltimore, including Dr. William Welch from Johns Hopkins Hospital, Holman received outside support for her endeavors to create the Holman Association for the Promotion of Rural Nursing, Hygiene, and Social Service. Along with financial support, the Carolina, Clinchfield and Ohio Railway provided property that included a little building, where Holman was able to establish a small hospital in Altapass, North Carolina. In her 1914–1915 informal report, included in the 1918 publication, Holman stated that the facility should be viewed not as a hospital but as

> a Settlement, with an infirmary. Our especial aim is to keep the family intact, and care for them at home unless we know they cannot recover there, when we bring them to the Infirmary. There is no part of family life we do not administer to [Holman, 1918, p. 3–4].

Holman was also in charge of the federal and state health programs when they became established in Mitchell County. She remained in Mitchell County until her death in 1960.

Neither Lydia Holman in North Carolina nor Mary Breckinridge of the Frontier Nursing Service in Kentucky were unique to visiting nursing and public health in these states. They reflected the dedication, creativity, perseverance, and resilience that was illustrative of the many pioneer public health nurses in the core of Appalachia and the difference these nurses made in bringing healthcare to the region.

District Health Departments and Public Health Nurses

Toward the middle of the twentieth century, district health departments gradually became established across the United States, including in each state of Southern Appalachia. Public health nurses were employed to administer community-wide programs aimed at

Appalachian Nursing

disease prevention; immunizations; school health; maternal, infant, and child health; and, in some regions, Native American health. Public health nurses served in various capacities where their responsibilities depended on the needs of the region and each state.

Grace McDaniels, Public Health Nurse, North Carolina

Grace McDaniels was the public health field nurse for the Qualla Boundary (official name for Cherokee-owned and -controlled land) in western North Carolina during the fiscal year of 1954–1955. In her annual report submitted to the Department of the Interior, Office of Indian Affairs Field Service, McDaniels described field nursing activities during the year. The Qualla Boundary had a population of 2,250 individuals residing in 400 homes that usually housed more than one family and were located off the roads, requiring her to walk a "considerable distance." She sometimes had to climb a mountain to conduct her visits. During 1954–1955, McDaniels made 274 home visits to 130 homes (most of which were small, with no windows or ventilation). Since most of these homes were located in the mountains, she found it difficult to reach many of the people who lived in the inaccessible areas. In an attempt to reach a larger number of residents in the region, McDaniels developed clinic centers that were conveniently located in each community. With easy access, residents gradually began to show interest in the clinics and attended a clinic when it was offered.

There were five schools on the Qualla Boundary. McDaniels performed physicals and immunizations at the individual schools. She found hygiene to be an issue, so most of her focus was directed toward school hygiene and sanitation. Malnutrition was another problem that needed to be addressed. McDaniels followed up with the children and also made prenatal and infant home visits. She held classes in home hygiene and care of the sick, in addition to providing classroom health talks. However, most of her work consisted of home visits for the children in the schools. McDaniel's main concerns were related to sanitation and infant mortality. Intestinal problems and diarrhea were prevalent. She conducted a sanitation survey of 93 homes, created folders for each family, and concluded her report with the suggestion that further sanitary supervision was needed on the Qualla Boundary (Jennings, n.d.).

III. Early Nursing Practice

Patty Norton, Public Health Nurse, Morgan County, West Virginia

Patty Norton lived in Hampshire County, West Virginia, just across the line from Morgan County. Born in Maryland, Norton graduated from the Allegheny Hospital School of Nursing in 1934 and moved to Pin Oak, West Virginia, after marrying her husband in 1936. In 1949, she became the Morgan County health nurse, and most of her work was carried out in the town of Magnolia. Norton recalled that at the time, the only telephone available in the town was a phone owned by the railroad and located in the home of the railroad foreman. There was no electricity in Magnolia, and the only access into and out of the town was by way of a single unpaved road that wound across steep mountain ridges and ended at the cemetery.

Norton held well-child clinics each month at a local resident's home, using the kitchen table for her equipment. Mothers and their children came to attend her clinics, some of them traveling from communities a far distance away, but as they had been raised in Magnolia, attending a clinic there gave them a chance to visit with family and friends. Norton provided free vitamins and health brochures, gave instructions for remedies and medications, passed out menus for healthy diets, and provided pre- and postnatal care, as well as instruction on prevention of communicable diseases. She also served as a nurse at the school in Paw Paw, another community in Morgan County, and kept Magnolia residents up to date with school activities. Norton, a friend to the community, retired in 1975 (Shambaugh, 2003).

Public Health Nursing and Trachoma

Trachoma, an eye disease that led to blindness, was a significant problem throughout the Appalachian region. Mae Hicks, a public health nurse in the mountains of eastern Kentucky, was chief nurse of the Trachoma Control Program in Kentucky. She and other public health nurses worked in trachoma clinics in their communities, but they also made home visits to follow up with patients, teaching about hygiene and proper sanitation (Kentucky Nurses Association, 2006).

Midwifery

In the core of Appalachia, as in other regions of the United States, midwifery played an important role in the healthcare of pregnant mothers during the eighteenth through the early twentieth centuries. Granny midwives (sometimes called "granny doctors" or "granny women") were common in most rural Southern Appalachian communities. In fact, they were usually the only source of maternal birthing assistance in the core of Appalachia prior to the introduction of the Frontier Nursing Service. As was the case in other rural areas across the United States, the community granny midwife provided a necessary service delivering babies in the rural and isolated communities of Appalachia where, due to the rugged mountainous geography, access to care was essentially nonexistent. In these communities, horseback was the primary form of transportation, and the granny midwife might well be the only source of medical help in the area. Occasionally the granny midwife would treat other members of the family or community who were sick or injured; however, her primary focus was to attend to the pregnant mothers in the delivery of their babies, referred to as "kotchin'" (or "catching babies").

Granny midwives typically had no formal midwifery training, nor were they professionally educated nurses, midwives, or doctors, and most could not read or write. They usually acquired their skills through personal experience with their own family, being present during other deliveries, apprenticing with an experienced granny midwife, or being chosen by an older midwife in their family to carry on that role. One older retired granny midwife shared that her mother, sister, and mother-in-law were all midwives (Scott 1982).

West Virginia Women's Commission (1983) pre- and postnatal care was not provided by the granny midwife. Most midwives treated their patients with folk medicine, including teas and herbs; they might also recite spells or use other traditional methods passed down from earlier generations, such as placing an axe under the bed to relieve hemorrhaging (Poole, 1932; Scott, 1982). Granny midwives commonly used catnip tea to facilitate the baby's first bowel movement or ensure nourishment in cases of an inadequate supply of mother's milk. To comfort or heal, castor oil was popular and also frequently used to hasten labor (Bickley, 1990; Scott, 1982).

In a 1917 article, Clara M. Davis (of Berea, Kentucky, who later became a physician) described a typical Berea County birthing

III. Early Nursing Practice

("kotching") as told to her by a visiting nurse who had been invited to experience the birth:

> Seated upon the lap of another woman was the expectant mother and in front of her, on another chair, was the old midwife. On either side of the midwife and holding the legs of the woman were two of the neighbors. Two more were supporting the knees of the "nuss." ... The woman was in the second stage of labor and the midwife sitting with knees close under the woman's hips, with hands and apron ready to "kotch the baby," was helping and encouraging, as midwives have done since the days of Pharaoh. Lacerations were not considered, the main object being to get the baby as quickly as possible.... The baby was "kotched," and its face wiped off with a corner of the apron. The placenta came presently and was likewise "kotched," then the midwife pushed back and gave the order, "Fotch on a piece of stout string so I can tie this cord" ... the family scissors were brought into the game, the placenta dropped to the floor and the baby, wrapped in the same useful apron, was handed to its waiting grandmother ... the old midwife had bathed ... the baby in the family wash basin, put on a cord dressing of scorched rags and "hog's fat," and dressed the mite in its first clothes [Davis, 1917, pp. 704–705].

In one survey of 84 midwives across Kentucky, West Virginia, Tennessee, North Carolina, and northern Georgia who practiced during the 1920s to 1930s, most (61) respondents were from Kentucky (Floyd, Knott, Leslie, McCreary, Owsley, and Pike counties), along with others who had worked or were currently working in West Virginia (2), Tennessee (1), North Carolina (13), and northern Georgia (7). All but three midwives surveyed in this study were white; 65 were married and 19 were widowed. Eighty-two of the midwives had borne children, 42 could not read or write, 66 learned midwifery by doing it, and 17 had learned by doing and also attended health department classes. Many of these granny midwives practiced in their own communities, serving their neighbors and relatives. For those who were paid in currency, the fee ranged from $3 to $5, whereas doctors would frequently charge $10–$30. Most of the patients could not afford a cash payment, and the midwives would often accept gifts, food, or sometimes favors (Scott, 1982).

Orlean (sometimes spelled Orleana or even Orelena) Puckett stands as an excellent example of the long-standing granny midwives who practiced in the core of Appalachia, providing a needed service to the community. Puckett never received any formal training as a midwife and could not read or write. Born 1844 in North Carolina, Orlean

Hawks married John Puckett at the age of 16, and they settled in Virginia (National Park Service, 2021). During the late 1800s, as was the case in many other isolated rural communities, there were very few doctors in Virginia's Carroll and Patrick counties. Due to the large geographic area to cover, doctors had little time to care for pregnant women or deliver babies. At the age of 45 years, Puckett filled that void. She lived in the area, and, despite her illiteracy, she was knowledgeable about folk remedies and cures. Puckett could also reach the residents more quickly than the doctor. She began her practice in 1889 when no doctor or other midwife could be located for a local neighbor in labor. Thus began Puckett's years of service in the community. Following that first birth, she became identified in the area as a midwife. Known for her capabilities and compassion, Puckett traveled across the region (sometimes journeying twenty miles at a time) to deliver babies. She went on to deliver more than 1,000 babies without loss of life to a baby or mother. Puckett was known to carry an old, brown leather doctor's bag (thought to have been given to her by one of the doctors). In the bag were scissors, gauze, twine, camphor, and eye drops. When delivering a baby, she would give the infant tea made from catnip with sugar before the mother's milk was in. She also used peach brandy for deliveries as well as for colds (Smith, 2003).

In addition to caring for the women giving birth, Puckett cared for other members of the family, never charging for her services. Instead, she would accept food from the family as payment. These offerings included items such as corn, beans, dried apples, cabbage, honey, hog meat, fatback, and sometimes coffee, ginger, or a live chicken. The local doctors were glad to have Puckett attend the births since, in most cases, they were not able to reach the mother when her labor began (Smith, 2003). Although she did not call herself a midwife, Puckett was referred to and known to the community residents as a midwife. She was highly respected and loved by the community. As with many other granny midwives, Puckett continued to practice well into her later life. Having spent 50 years as a granny midwife in the region, Orlean Puckett died in 1939. As a tribute to her legacy, the Orleana Hawks Puckett Institute was created in Asheville, North Carolina, to promote child, parent, and family development. In addition, Puckett was posthumously honored at the Library of Virginia as one of the Virginia Women in History ("Orleana Hawks Puckett," 2012).

In 1921, the Sheppard-Towner Act was established to provide

III. Early Nursing Practice

funds for the healthcare of mothers and infants. The purpose was to address mortality rates among mothers and newborn infants, and $1 million of federal aid per year was provided to state programs, specifically for prenatal care to mothers and their newborn babies in rural states. This act also began regulation of the practice of midwifery. Regulation, however, was slow to evolve in the Appalachian region. For example, in a 1922 report of births to the Health Department for Leslie, Knott and Owsley counties in east Kentucky, there were a total of 9 doctors and 128 midwives. Of 968 births, 824 were attended by midwives and 144 by doctors. One doctor in the region emphasized that there remained a significant need for midwives: "We absolutely cannot do without them ... the midwife is a necessity here" (Breckinridge, 1923, p. 13).

In 1925, midwifery became state regulated. Regulation required midwives to be trained, licensed, and registered. In 1926, it was mandated that no one other than a physician could practice as a midwife without being licensed. Individual states then set their own standards for licensure. For example, the West Virginia Department of Health required applicants to be able to read and write and possess a diploma from a school of midwifery or a doctor's statement certifying that she had attended five births (Bickley, 1990). In 1938, West Virginia's health department began providing its own midwifery training.

Even though state regulation and the Sheppard-Towner Act had been established, there were no formal midwifery services provided by trained nurse midwives until the Frontier Nursing Service was established in 1925. Even then, granny midwives continued to provide their services in the rural, isolated areas of Appalachia well into the mid-twentieth century. These granny midwives were usually members of the community who had practiced through multiple generations of families. They were well loved and trusted. Although state regulation mandated professional education and registration, many of these granny midwives chose not to pursue additional training or state approval, and they continued to practice through word of mouth.

With the assistance of a midwife, home births were popular in the core of Appalachia and remained a common tradition as late as the 1940s/1950s. Similar to a quilting bee or corn-shucking gathering, they frequently served as a social time for neighbors to get together.

Appalachian Nursing

Frontier Nursing Service—The Early Years of Professionalism in Midwifery

One of most well-known midwifery and visiting nurses' services in the United States is the Frontier Nursing Service (FNS), an iconic example of nurses who traveled on horseback across rivers and rugged mountains to bring maternal and child healthcare to their patients in Kentucky. The FNS, established in 1925, is one of two nurse-managed organizations in the United States that was founded by a nurse (in this case, Mary Breckinridge) and is still in existence today. The other nurse-managed organization was the Henry Street Settlement in New York City founded by Lillian Wald in 1893. Although there were more than thirty years between the establishment of the Frontier Nursing Service and the Henry Street Settlement, there were similarities between these organizations and the nurses who created them. Despite the geographical distance and three-decade difference in development and establishment of the two nursing organizations, both Breckinridge and Wald sought to bring desperately needed healthcare to communities with limited resources. One organization (the Henry Street Settlement) was in the middle of a large city with many physicians and hospitals. The other (Frontier Nursing Service) was located in a rugged, isolated region many miles away from any doctor or hospital. Despite being in distinctly different regions of the United States, these two nurse-led organizations had something in common: they were established to address the lack of access to healthcare for a very poor or isolated population unable to obtain medical assistance either inside or outside of their community. The Henry Street Settlement brought healthcare to a poor immigrant community in New York City, while the Frontier Nursing Service brought midwifery and nursing care to residents in the remote rural region of eastern Kentucky. Both Wald and Breckinridge had strong work ethics; they were proponents for precise recordkeeping and evaluation of their organization's work. In addition, Wald and Breckinridge had a strong desire to help those less fortunate with limited access to healthcare. They also had the benefit of connections with high-ranking individuals and organizations for funding and support.

Mary Breckinridge was born in Memphis, Tennessee, to an affluent and influential family that had ancestral roots in Kentucky. Her grandfather, John C. Breckinridge, had been vice president to President James

III. Early Nursing Practice

Buchanan, and her father served in Congress. As a privileged young girl living in Washington, D.C., Breckinridge grew up in comfort, and it was through her father's work in government that she became aware of issues that impacted rural areas of the country. As Breckinridge matured into adulthood, she maintained an interest in rural health issues, and it expanded to include the needs of mothers and children in isolated communities. As a young girl, however, Breckinridge was not interested in nursing; she married at the age of 23 and became a widow two years later. After her husband's death, she began to consider what she wanted to do with her life and made the decision to become a nurse. Breckinridge entered the nurses' training program at St. Luke's Hospital in New York City and graduated in 1910. However, she did not practice immediately; instead, shortly after graduation, she married again. Her second marriage produced two children who both died very young. After several miscarriages, and a difficult marriage, Breckinridge eventually divorced her second husband (Breckinridge, 1952; Poole, 1932). The unexpected early deaths of her two children were hard on Breckinridge, which became central in her subsequent dedication to the health and welfare of children. In her biography, Breckinridge reflected on the death of her son, Breckie:

> God ... cherishes them there, and I fight for them—fight until that ancient saying has come true, until He shall gather the Lambs ... in his bosom, and gently lead those that are with young. And when the crooked paths are made straight and the waste places smooth it will be time enough for me to understand [Breckinridge, 1952, p. 74].

These words would ultimately become the motto for the Frontier Nursing Service.

In 1918, Breckinridge joined the American Committee for Devastated France to help those who were starving in French villages. While working with the French midwives, she observed that midwives in France were not trained nurses, just as nurses trained in the United States were not midwives; however, in England, trained nurses also served as midwives. Breckinridge concluded that trained nurse midwives would be a logical way to address the health of children in the United States. She believed that in the United States, children in the more urban regions and cities were mostly taken care of because of access to resources, but those in the isolated, rural areas of the country were neglected. Breckinridge was convinced that the work for children should begin before birth with a comprehensive focus on the first six years of their lives. She decided her work would best be carried out in the remote and rural areas of the United States, where it was needed the most. She was also aware of the additional education in public health that was required for her to be effective in her efforts to bring healthcare to the Kentucky mountains. She likewise knew that she needed to learn more about conditions in the remote areas of Kentucky, her ancestral homeplace.

Breckinridge returned to the United States and began to plan for her life's work in helping children get the best start in life from birth. She spent a year immersing herself in public health and corresponding coursework at Teachers College, Columbia University, in New York. During the summer of 1923, Breckinridge conducted a survey with the assistance of three nurses (Edna Rockstroh, Freida Caffin, and Bertram Ireland) focusing on the conditions of midwifery across three counties in Kentucky. The nurses met with local residents to learn firsthand about the conditions and needs within the region. In addition, Breckinridge visited Scotland in 1924 and met with Sir Leslie Mackenzie, chief medical officer of the Highlands and Islands Medical Nursing Service (HIMNS), to learn more about the organization, since that region of Scotland had similar socioeconomic and geographical conditions to those that prevailed in eastern Kentucky. Breckinridge became friends with Mackenzie and his wife, Lady Mackenzie. Because of the quality of the HIMNS program in Scotland, as well as its similarity to the issues and conditions in eastern Kentucky, Breckinridge returned to Kentucky and adapted the FNS midwifery program to the HIMNS template. Aware that she also needed formal midwife training, Breckinridge went back to Europe to study midwifery at the British Hospital for Mothers and Babies (Campbell, 1984). She successfully completed the midwifery training program in Britain, passed the certification examination under the central Midwives Board in London, and became what was referred to as "an American certificated English Midwife" (Breckinridge, 1952, p. 129). Breckinridge returned to Kentucky early in 1925 with a strong belief that nurse midwifery was a way to address the health of young children, especially those neglected in the remote areas of the United States. In her autobiography, Breckinridge described her early thoughts as she left England:

> Something else is mine to do back in my own land. I don't know what yet, but I dream dreams and see visions and the dreams.... I know that the way leads back over the ocean to the country where my own children were born [Breckinridge, 1952, p. 95].

III. Early Nursing Practice

Breckinridge was determined to focus her efforts on the rural regions of the United States, as she felt strongly that children in these areas were more likely to be neglected than those who lived in cities. Considering the poverty and lack of access to healthcare for residents in the remote Kentucky mountains, Breckinridge wanted to establish a nursing service in that region. Her vision was that, if successful, the work could be duplicated in other isolated areas of the United States.

A country doctor from Owsley County, Kentucky, shared with Breckinridge that he could not possibly reach every family in the remote areas of the region. He said that in some cases it could take a doctor six to twenty hours by horseback to reach a patient and told Breckinridge the local granny midwives provided a necessary service, as "it is impossible for me to reach every hoot-owl hollow in my section in time to be of any use to a woman in childbirth. Midwives are essential here." The doctor also felt that professional training of the midwives would be beneficial: "I wish they might be nurses as well" (Breckinridge, 1952, p. 229).

After she returned from England, Breckinridge quickly set out to establish the first demonstration project of nurse midwifery in the Kentucky Mountains. Dr. Arthur McCormack, health commissioner of Kentucky, approved of Breckinridge's plan. He also awarded Breckinridge a license to practice as a midwife in Kentucky. Organized in May 1925, what was to eventually become the Frontier Nursing Service (FNS) was originally named the Kentucky Committee for Mothers and Babies. The model of this new nursing organization was based on Breckinridge's work in France, as well as the HIMNS, and it also reflected her philosophy, experience, and training. Its purpose was

> to safeguard the lives and health of mothers and young children by providing trained nurse-midwives for rural areas where there are no resident physicians—these nurse midwives to work under supervision; in compliance with the Regulations for Midwives of the State Board of Health, and the law governing the Registration of Nurses in Kentucky; and in co-operation with the nearest medical service [Kentucky Committee for Mothers and Babies, 1926, p. 1].

The motto Breckinridge selected for her new organization illustrated the impact her son Breckie's death had on her: "He shall gather the lambs with his arm and carry them in his bosom, and shall gently lead those that are with young" (Breckinridge, 1952, p. 74).

With a clear vision and plan, combined with her experience in

Appalachian Nursing

France and Scotland, ancestral family roots, and high-ranking connections in Kentucky, Breckinridge operationalized her plan for a midwifery service in the rural Kentucky mountains. She believed the best organizational approach in this isolated region would be through decentralization of the midwifery service, with establishment of a central clinic and nursing outpost centers. The proposed service would include midwifery, public health, and bedside nursing. Nurses hired for the Frontier Nursing Service were required to be properly trained in midwifery. Although there was a small midwifery training school in New York City, the Maternity Center Association, Breckinridge felt the best midwifery education was located in England and Scotland, and the HIMNS rural model was in better alignment with the Kentucky region and population served by the FNS. Most of the midwifery nurses originally hired for service in the FNS came from England and Scotland, where they received their midwifery training. American nurses hired for the FNS were required to have received midwifery training and graduation from a recognized midwifery program. After a successful six-month probation period with the Frontier Nursing Service, the American nurses without formal midwifery training were sent to England for training that was fully paid for by the Frontier Nursing Service. After successful completion of the English midwifery program and receipt of a midwifery license, the nurses then returned to the United States to complete a course in public health, at which point they became official frontier nurses. In addition, every new nurse received riding lessons, since horses and mules were the only source of transportation available to the FNS in the core region of Appalachia (Breckinridge, 1952).

The FNS concept of decentralization was the result of addressing geography and weather issues. It was based on the amount of travel time (instead of mileage) needed to reach a patient from each outpost center. Using this approach, the farthest patient could be reached within an hour during good weather. During bad weather, such as a blizzard, it could take two or more hours to reach the patient. Each outpost was to be located in the center of a five-mile radius, approximately nine to twelve miles apart. Where the territory for one nurse midwife ended, another began. The outposts were geographically placed following waterways since that was the main form of travel and trade in the remote areas of the region. The outposts were to be built along two main rivers: the middle fork of the Kentucky River,

III. Early Nursing Practice

the Red Bird River, and tributaries. Aided by donations from national sources and support from the community, physicians, local authorities, and others, the Kentucky Committee for Mothers and Babies was established in September 1925 with the opening of its first central clinic in Hyden, Kentucky. Wendover, the administrative headquarters (and Breckinridge's residence), was the next clinic, established in March 1926; the Jessie Preston Draper Center, known as Beech Fork Clinic, then opened in October of that same year (Breckinridge, 1952).

HYDEN CENTER

The Hyden Center was opened with two nurse midwives, Edna Rockstroh and Freida Caffin, whom Breckinridge had met while in England. Both Rockstroh and Caffin received their midwifery training at Queen Charlotte's Hospital in London. In a 1979 interview, Rockstroh recalled the midwifery training at Queen Charlotte's as strict but a "good experience." To complete the program, nurses were required to deliver (under supervision) 50 babies in the hospital, followed by another 30 babies in the community setting (Rockstroh, 1979).

At the Hyden Center, the nurse midwives' territory covered 78 square miles, with midwifery, public health, and bedside nursing care provided to approximately one thousand residents. By the end of the first year, 70 pregnant women had registered, prenatal care was provided, and 40 babies had been successfully delivered. In that first year Rockstroh and Caffin also provided vaccinations against typhoid and diphtheria to the region's residents. They traveled as far as a day's ride away to care for patients with typhoid who lived beyond the center's district. When asked whether she and Caffin had any difficulty gaining acceptance in the community, Rockstroh responded "no," explaining that they first visited the families in the community, let the residents know they were trained midwives, and provided details about the services they could provide to the community (Rockstroh, 1979).

Rockstroh talked about the idea of a trading post at Hyden. Caffin's mother, Caroline Caffin, while developing a public health association in 1926 and visiting her daughter Freida at the Hyden Center, had expanded on the idea of opening a trading post there. She had many friends in New York and wrote to them asking that they ship clothing of all kinds (including shoes, stockings, coats, and toys) to the Hyden

House Clinic. She then conducted a "trade day" twice a week, at which time the residents would bring corn, chicken, and eggs to trade for the clothes and other items. The residents enjoyed the time they spent at these gatherings, during which they could sit around, talk to each other and "gossip." The nurses likewise enjoyed the fresh food.

In her interview, Rockstroh described the Hyden Center as a model. It was the first one of its kind located in the Leslie County seat and also served as the nursing supervisor's headquarters. Both Rockstroh and Caffin had their own district for which they were responsible. Rockstroh described the role of the nurses. Each nurse midwife was provided with a horse, a saddle, and saddle bags. The saddle bags contained essential supplies for both nursing and deliveries. For general nursing, the bags included cotton bandages, tongue depressors, vaccines, and materials for urinalysis. In order to prevent breakage, medications were placed in cans. Bags for deliveries also included a rubber sheet and five enamel basins. The packed bags weighed 38 pounds, and items were equally distributed between the two bags. The delivery bags weighed an additional 10 pounds. The nurses also carried a lantern for light when traveling in the dark and snake serum to be used for rattlesnake and copperhead bites (Poole, 1932).

WENDOVER CENTER

The opening of the Wendover Center came in March 1926, and it was patterned after the program pioneered at Hyden. While the area was similar in size to Hyden, the population was much smaller, and there was one nurse in charge: Ellen Halsall. Wendover was also the administrative center, with a guest house and residence for Breckinridge. There were many travelers from long distances who visited Wendover, including Annette Dohring (a nurse from the American Committee for Devastated France who was on a scholarship to study the methods of Breckinridge's organization).

THE JESSIE PRESTON DRAPER CENTER

The Jessie Preston Draper Center opened around October 1926. It was located at the mouth of Bad Creek, near where the Beech Fork and Middle Fork rivers converged (thus leading to its alternate name of the Beech Fork Clinic). Gladys Peacock and Mary B. Willeford were the first nurses to open the district and staff the center. There had been some

III. Early Nursing Practice

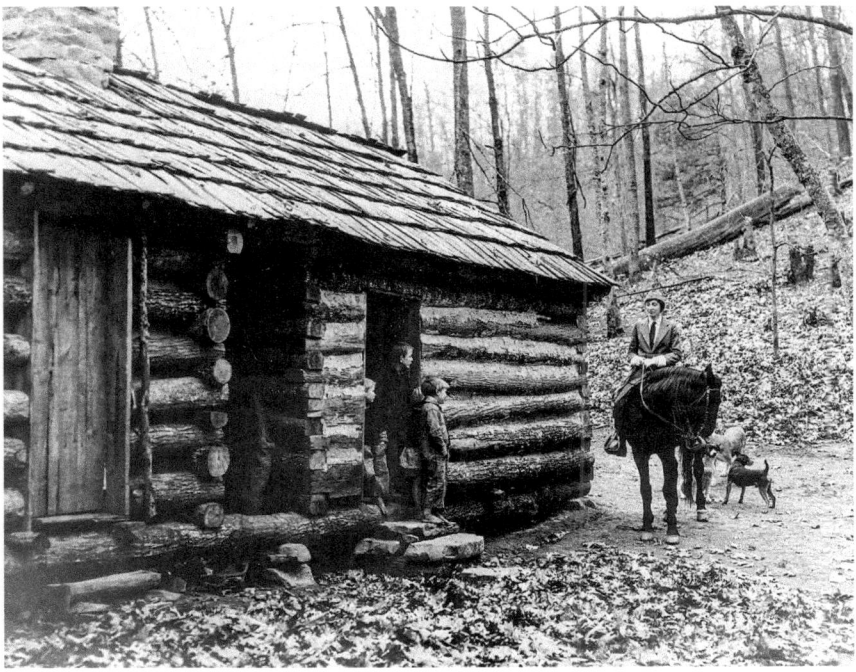

Visiting nurse in Kentucky backwoods: "Friend, Nurse and Counsellor—a member of the Pioneer Nursing Service calls upon a lonely home in the Kentucky mountains" (Associated Press Photo, New York, December 2, 1932).

difficulty in finding someone to construct the center building itself, so volunteers stepped in. It took a team of workers three days and nights to get to the railroad and return with supplies. Residents of the community donated wood, along with their time and effort, to help build the center (Kentucky Committee for Mothers and Babies, 1925).

Both Peacock and Willeford were promoted to assistant directors of the FNS and received furloughs to further their education at Teachers College, Columbia University, in New York City. Peacock earned her BS degree and Willeford a PhD in educational research. They both returned to the FNS in the summer of 1932. Willeford's research focused on a study of 400 families in remote rural areas of Leslie County, Kentucky, in which she wrote about the region and the patients served. The results were published in the January 1933 issue of the *American Journal of Nursing* (Willeford, 1933).

Appalachian Nursing

HYDEN HOSPITAL

In addition to the clinics, Breckinridge soon recognized the need for a hospital in the region. There was a consistent concern when emergencies arose due to the difficulties of reaching a doctor combined with the many hours it could take for a doctor to arrive when needed. To make matters worse, the closest hospital was more than thirty miles away over rough terrain. Breckinridge decided that once the Hyden Center was open, she would begin thinking about plans for a hospital in the region.

Two obstetrical emergencies (placenta previa) arose during the summer of 1927 that clearly indicated the significant need for a hospital to be established as soon as possible. In both emergency situations, the nurses had to send for a physician. In one case, it took over three days and four attempts spanning four counties before a physician arrived, as two of the physicians were on holiday, and one could not come; finally, the last doctor, J.P. Boggs of Hazard County, agreed to make the 33-mile trip at night on horseback. In that particular case, the family was not aware of the seriousness of the patient's condition and would not have known to summon a doctor. Credit was given to the nurse midwife service, suggesting that if it had not been for the midwife quickly recognizing the problem and locating a doctor, the patient could have died. The baby did not survive, but the mother did. In the second case, the nurse took care of the patient until the doctor arrived several hours after having been summoned. Both mother and baby survived. Dr. Boggs, the physician, praised the nurse:

> I sure was glad to hear about both patients getting so much better. Also was glad to find Mrs. ——— better when I got there. If Miss Caffin had not had the nerve to plunge and take hold she would have been a dead patient by the time I got there. So we certainly have to commend her for her bravery, and I think she deserves a medal more so than Lindbergh [Boggs, 1927, p. 4].

As a result of these cases, Breckinridge decided that a hospital with a medical director whose services could be readily relied on was essential. In addition, she and the midwives could plan in advance for medical coverage. Breckinridge commenced making plans for a twelve-bed hospital in Hyden. The hospital plans also included living quarters for the nurses and district midwives. Generous donations and individual gifts, along with financial support from the state of Kentucky, helped to build and furnish the hospital. By mid–1928, Hyden Hospital was

III. Early Nursing Practice

close to completion. There were two wards with four beds each, space for the same number of children's beds, and space for 25 patients in special clinics. The hospital had an operating room with supplies, a dispensary, a waiting room, a kitchen, supply rooms, and baths. There was also a laboratory for the county health director. The nurses of the district, supervisor, and bookkeeper likewise had sleeping quarters.

On June 26, 1928, Hyden Hospital was formally opened and dedicated. Since the Frontier Nursing Service had been modeled after the Highlands and Islands Medical Nursing Service in Scotland, led by Sir Leslie Mackenzie (whom Breckinridge had met during her time in Europe), Breckinridge felt it was fitting for Mackenzie to deliver the dedication address for Hyden Hospital. Mackenzie and his wife accepted Breckinridge's invitation and traveled from Scotland to attend the dedication. In his speech, Mackenzie talked about the similarities between the two organizations and the needs of what he called the "thinly populated people," describing those living in rural, isolated areas:

> When some years ago, Mrs. Mary Breckinridge came to us in Scotland to see how we faced a similar problem in medical service and nursing, we were filled with a new sense of the significance of the work we had tried to do in the thinly peopled and difficult areas of Scotland. I felt indeed, a glow of supreme satisfaction that our work in Scotland had found an echo in the great spaces and mountains of an American Commonwealth.... From my earliest memories, I have known something of the difficulties of Highland life, and when I passed into the National Service I came to the health problems of the Highlands and Islands with some understanding of the inner minds and aspirations of the people, of the difficulties, due to a long and losing struggle with poverty and of the problems created by centuries of European invasion.... In one respect, the problem of the Kentucky mountains is essentially the same as the problem of the Scottish Highlands and Islands— namely, that the financial resources of the thinly peopled areas are rarely, if ever, sufficient to provide the same adequate services that the larger groups of population enjoy. That was the root of our problem in Scotland. It is the root of the problem in the Commonwealth of Kentucky.... Wherever we find the thinly populated islands or mountains, there we find difficulty in providing sufficient services.... This hospital is the radiating centre of the nursing service in these mountains.... The hospital is a temple of service where the lamp never goes out.... Here in this temple of humanism, every hour is filled with a clear ideal. The mothers and fathers know that here they have friends that they can come to and speak to and live with. Through these mountains and forests, the Frontier Nursing Service will become a gracious presence transfiguring the individual lives.... The service draws its life from

Appalachian Nursing

an unfailing fountain of human sympathy and love. They will always feel that here on the frontier outposts, they are living out the true purpose of the Commonwealth—to prepare a worthy and dignified place for every child born to it....

In all reverence, I dedicate this hospital to the services of this mountain people.... Far in the future ... generation after generation, will arise to bless the name of the Frontier Nursing Service [Mackenzie, 1928, pp. 3–8].

Shortly after Hyden Hospital was dedicated, Breckinridge assigned Ann MacKinnon, a nurse from the Beech Fork Center, to the position of hospital superintendent. Dr. H.C. Capps was the medical director. Patients finally had a place to go during times of serious illness and injury. There were frequent burn cases among children, especially little girls whose skirts would get caught in the open fires that were common in people's homes. Patients arrived by mule, horseback, or stretcher (sometimes made by coats with poles run through the sleeves). Transporting a patient by stretcher over such great distances required sixteen volunteer carriers working in relays of four, with one person at the head, another at the foot and two on each side (Breckinridge, 1952).

As early as 1930, Hyden Hospital was well established and the FNS had grown from three to six outposts in the region. By 1932, the FNS had gained national recognition from public health leaders for the work and service provided in Kentucky. C.E.A. Winslow, a public health expert who founded the Department of Public Health at Yale, wrote:

One of the gravest handicaps under which the rural area has suffered has been the lack of elementary facilities for health protection. Doctors, dentists, nurses, hospitals, are almost non-existent over large areas; and lowered vitality spells economic backwardness.... The Frontier Nursing Service has shown us how this need can be met. I have studied Mrs. Breckinridge's records. I have visited the centers. I have ridden over the trails with her nurses. I can testify that the work is sound and that its administration is economical. The service has brought to the people of this Forgotten Frontier the alleviation of suffering, the prevention of needless disease, the safeguarding of motherhood, the possibility of health and happy children. The significance of this demonstration extends far beyond the confines of four Kentucky counties. It is a model for this country and for other countries. It is an enterprise of which the whole United States may be justly proud.... Its work must be preserved and carried forward [Winslow, 1932, p. 10; Frontier Nursing Service Primer 1932, p. 10].

By 1935, the FNS outposts had expanded to eight and became well known across the United States, Canada, and Europe. A sense

III. Early Nursing Practice

of adventure brought many nurses to the FNS from states far beyond Appalachia as well as Canada and other countries in Europe. As part of an oral history interview, one nurse midwife was asked why she came all the way to Kentucky from Canada: "I have a little bit of pioneer sense of adventure, I guess.... I had always thought about being ... a nurse in a rural area, and certainly what. I learned about the Frontier Nursing Service sounded like the right place" (Fee, 2002, p. 1).

In a 1939 report, Breckinridge described the Frontier Nursing Service as an adaptation of the Scottish Highland and Islands Medical and Nursing Service: "Our service was set up as a bit of international cooperation in this manner, and for years the staff was composed half of British and half of American nurses who had received their midwifery training in Great Britain" (Breckinridge, 1939, p. 24). For some time, Breckinridge had been considering the possibility of midwifery training in connection with the FNS. A large portion of the American nurses who were hired for the FNS did not have formal midwifery training, and within the first six months of being hired, they were sent to Great Britain to complete their training. The FNS initially provided scholarships to cover the costs of training, travel, housing, books and meals, and the nurses were allowed one year to complete their studies (Breckinridge, 1952). By 1939, however, the training costs for American nurses had become a significant financial issue for the FNS; scholarships to send the American nurses to Great Britain for midwifery training were eliminated, which had a negative impact on FNS staffing to the extent that the formally educated nurse midwives from Great Britain soon outnumbered the American nurses. The midwifery staff was two-thirds British nurses to one-third American nurses. It soon became necessary to consider establishing a midwifery training school for the FNS (Training Frontier Nurse-Midwives, 1939).

Frontier Nursing Service Midwifery Training School

As prologue to establishing the FNS Midwifery Training School, and at the request of the National Society of Colonial Dames in 1935, the Frontier Nursing Service accepted two Philadelphia-trained Native American nurses for a year's postgraduate work and experience in midwifery. The purpose of this training was to prepare these nurses to work on reservations in Wyoming and Nevada. The Colonial Dames

Appalachian Nursing

in Kentucky and the National Society of Colonial Dames in Massachusetts, Maine, and Michigan provided full scholarships for the two nurses. In addition to midwifery, the nurses were exposed to public health and nursing in the home setting. The Indian Bureau had plans to expand this service to other reservations in the Southwest for the purpose of providing medical and nurse midwifery services to the reservations (Breckinridge, 1952). One of the issues that became apparent in the training of the two nurses was the additional burden placed on the supervisory staff of the FNS, as the staff could not include additional training of graduate nurses with their regular responsibilities; more staff members were needed.

In 1939, the declaration of war in Europe had an additional impact on the FNS when the British nurses had to leave the United States and return home to serve their own country and war efforts. The departure of these nurse midwives created an emergency for the FNS and an immediate need for professionally trained nurse midwives to replace those who had left. It also served as the impetus to move forward with Breckinridge's plans for a midwifery training school so that the work of the FNS could continue. Breckinridge began by obtaining approval from the executive committee, with endorsement from the Medical Advisory Committee, the Kentucky State Board of Health, and community residents in the region served by the FNS (Annual Report, 1940). In addition, Breckinridge contacted Isabel Stewart and Lillian Hudson in the Nursing Department at Teachers College, Columbia University, to discuss the new midwifery course and ensure that it would meet Teachers College transfer credit guidelines for students who wished to pursue a BS degree (Training Frontier Nurse-Midwives, 1939).

Because of the similarity between Kentucky and the Scottish Highlands, Breckinridge made a visit to Scotland so that she could learn more about midwifery education at the Highlands and Island Medical and Nursing Service. Using their excellent program as an example, Breckinridge created the FNS midwifery training school. The FNS midwifery education followed the same methods and guidelines set by the Central Midwives' Boards of England and Scotland. Students were required to deliver 20 midwifery cases, including five in the hospital and five in the community. The practical teaching of students in the hospital was conducted by Betty Lester, FNS assistant hospital superintendent; the community cases were taught by Nora Kelly, FNS assistant director. Both women were graduates of well-regarded English midwifery

III. Early Nursing Practice

schools. The FNS midwifery lectures were given by Dr. Kooser, and the periodic examinations were administered by Dorothy Buck. The training was focused on managing normal conditions, preventing and recognizing the abnormal, and, if necessary, applying emergency procedures before the arrival of the physician. Instruction would include knowledge of general health and risks during childbearing, practice in abdominal exams, external pelvimetry, urinalysis, and blood pressure. Students received instruction in physiology, management and progress of labor, and care of the mother and newborn baby. Prenatal and postpartum experience would be provided in the home and specialty midwifery clinics in the hospital. Each student would make prenatal visits and have a caseload of patients from birth until the baby was nine months old (Buck, D., 1940).

Breckinridge had a strong connection to New York and established a collaboration between the FNS and the Lobenstine Clinic in New York City. Under the auspices of the Maternity Center Association, the Lobenstine Clinic agreed to take FNS students for part of their midwifery practicum experience. Scholarships, gifts from the FNS trustees, were provided for training of the first five students in the program. (In addition, there was a benefactor in Ohio who donated money for training equipment, books and bookcases.) The FNS Graduate School of Midwifery officially opened on November 1, 1939, with two students (Breckinridge, 1952).

Missions and Settlement Schools

The home and settlement movement made its way to Southern Appalachia during the late nineteenth to mid-twentieth centuries. Some of the settlements were religion based, while others were based on the concept of social service needs that originally emerged from the Hull House in Chicago. (Hull House was a settlement house founded by Jane Addams that brought education and social services to immigrants in Chicago.) Whether religion or social service based, the settlement movement in Appalachia had a similar goal—namely, providing educational and social service resources to isolated communities in Appalachia. Church boards across a variety of faiths recognized a need for missionary work, education, social services, and healthcare in the remote communities of Southern Appalachia. Access to public schools and social resources was limited or nonexistent in some areas of the region. Each home mission board provided services that were tailored to each specific community, depending on its needs. Although the primary goal of most settlement schools was to provide education to children and resources to the families in the region, the lack of healthcare in the remote rural communities was clearly evident. If not an original focus of those organizations, healthcare resources and services were frequently incorporated into the settlement so that residents of the community had access to healthcare in addition to education and social services (Campbell, 1921).

Hindman, Kentucky

Hindman Settlement School, established in 1902 in Knott County, Kentucky, was one of the first rural social settlements in the United States. The original funding came from the Women's Christian Temperance Union, and the purpose was to establish educational programs and address a number of social and health-related needs in the community (Stoddart, 2002). In 1905, Harriet Butler was hired as the nurse for the Hindman Settlement School, and she established a program of health education, home visits, and physical exams for the students. In addition, she helped with the plans to build a hospital in connection with the settlement. Her work extended to treating residents in the community and had expanded to the extent that another nurse was hired for rural nursing and health education to address the needs of the community. In 1915, the settlement sponsored a Red Cross nurse and trained two additional Red Cross nurses for visiting nursing in the community. Nurses provided healthcare for residents in the county as a partnership between Knott County and Hindman Settlement. Trachoma, an eye disease that causes blindness, had spread across Appalachia. The nurses helped Dr. J. Stucky with his trachoma clinics, which were successful in the early intervention and treatment of the disease (Fighting Trachoma in Kentucky, 1914).

In addition to trachoma and other communicable diseases, nurses provided children's health examinations in schools. By 1917, over one thousand children throughout Knott County had received a health examination at their school. During the 1920s, Hindman's community nursing service was turned over to the county, with a nursing staff maintained on their physical site until 1967 (Stoddart, 2002).

III. Early Nursing Practice

Red Bird, Beverly, Kentucky

Red Bird (known as the Kentucky Mountain Mission of the United Methodist Church) was established in 1921 in Beverly, Kentucky. The goal of the Methodist Church was to provide education, socioeconomic assistance and Christian evangelism to the community residents. Red Bird began under the Board of Missions of the Evangelical Church, merged with the United Brethren Church, and later united with the Methodist Church as a school for the community. The Beverly community was located in a remote and very rural area of Kentucky, and, in addition to education and socioeconomic assistance, access to medical care was a significant need. Teachers and a minister were the first to arrive at Red Bird. The Reverend Dewall was the minister and superintendent assigned to the mission. On arrival, he noted the community residents lacked access to healthcare and were at risk for illness. Dewall also found that most of the residents used methods that he referred to as being superstitious and crude, sometimes worse than the disease they were trying to cure.

Healthcare services began in 1922 when Miss Lydia Rice, RN, from Nebraska arrived at Red Bird Mission after responding to a notice from the Board of Missions of the Evangelical Church. Rice took care of not only the Red Bird staff but also residents of the community and surrounding area. She was the only nurse/medical provider at the mission and traveled by mule to care for families in the rugged mountains of Bell County, treating illnesses, setting broken bones, and tending to other problems (including bullet wounds). Rice was frequently called out at all hours and described one call on a Sunday when the husband came for her. She followed him on her mule, traveling 12 miles through the mountains to reach his home. As Rice told the story afterward, "It was raining, the creeks were swollen, water was rushing noisily.... I couldn't see or hear my guide ... we stopped at a cabin for a carbide lamp ... the patient died a few hours after we arrived" (Kentucky Nurses Association, 2006, p. 33). Although she had been hired to take charge of the mission's medical work, Rice also embarked on education and sanitation for the community. Her approach to health was to keep the body physically fit in order to do the work of Christ. The goal was not only to care for the ill but also to focus on prevention. Rice taught the children to follow basic health rules and ensured that balanced diets were provided for the students.

Appalachian Nursing

In the Reverend Dewall's first annual report, he stated, "Our nurse, Miss Rice, though here but a short time, is receiving frequent calls and is bringing healing to both the body and the soul" (Weinert, 1959, p. 35).

The year 1923 brought the need for additional medical assistance that required a physician. Individuals required surgery; one was a woman from the community who could not be cured without surgical intervention. Her procedure was performed in the school building's Knuckles Hall by a visiting doctor who was a friend of the Reverend Dewall. The following week, a teacher required an appendectomy, which, again, was performed by the visiting doctor. Knuckles Hall became known as a hospital ward, and both incidents confirmed that Red Bird needed a resident doctor as well as a nurse. While the community searched for a resident doctor, they decided to begin offering "clinics" with the assistance of visiting doctors and nurses in 1925. The clinics were held two days at a time at various locations. In May 1925, one clinic was held in Beverly. Three doctors and two registered nurses, plus the mission nurse, were present at the clinic. Within two days, seventy patients had been examined, thirty-four surgeries were performed (including tonsillectomies on students at the mission) and twenty patients were also fitted for glasses. In 1926, Dr. Harlan Heim, a medical missionary who had served his internship at Bellevue Hospital in New York City, arrived at Red Bird as the resident physician. Rice, who had been well accepted in the community, helped dispel concerns about a new doctor whom the residents did not know and who was coming from New York City. By the end of the first month, 262 patients had been treated by the new doctor.

After Dr. Heim's arrival, it soon became clear that a hospital was needed at Red Bird. In 1928, a hospital was built for the community (Schaeffer, 1980). However, even after the hospital had opened, Rice and the staff continued to make home visits to residents in the community. By 1929, a total of 5,915 treatments had been provided to patients, and by 1930, there were 888 home visits (Red Bird Mission, n.d.).

In addition, a strong collaborative relationship had become established between the Red Bird Evangelical Hospital settlement and the Frontier Nursing Service by 1930. Mary Breckinridge mentioned this connection in her 1931 annual report when she stated that the FNS had maintained a relationship with the Presbyterian Center at Hyden for several years and had recently established a connection with an evangelical hospital settlement (more commonly known as the Red Bird Mission) located in Beverly, Bell County, Kentucky. Breckinridge assigned

III. Early Nursing Practice

Ellen Marsh ("Marshie," an FNS nurse midwife) to the Red Bird Mission. Marsh had completed the Queen's Nurses midwifery course in Edinburgh, Scotland, in early 1931, and her role with the Red Bird Mission was to work under Dr. Harlan Heim and cover his routine maternity cases. This assignment gave Heim the opportunity to increase his clinical services beyond Red Bird, to include the Jessie Preston Draper Center (Beech Fork) in Leslie County and the Carolina Butler Atwood Center (Flat Creek) in Clay County, Kentucky. It was an entire day's ride to each center, where Heim was (and remained) the only local physician for the area. Breckinridge concluded in her report that the association between the FNS and the Red Bird Mission was mutually beneficial (Breckinridge, 1952; Cooperation, 1931). Heim was impressed with Marsh and her work at the Red Bird Mission to the extent he wrote in a letter to the FNS, stating:

> It has been my intention to write you for a long time to tell you how very nicely Miss Marsh is doing.... She has become one of us so thoroughly that I cannot see how we ever did without her. The only thing I fear about her is that she does too much.... I realize now that her services are indispensable.... I express the thought of our workers here and a large number of the people of the community when I state that we are very grateful for her presence, and thankful to you for sending her to us [Cooperation, 1931, p. 15].

In addition to Marsh, two other nurses joined the Red Bird Mission nursing staff around the same time: Ruby Swisher from Ohio and Margaret Patterson from Illinois. By 1932, Rice had been appointed superintendent of the hospital. She remained at Red Bird for twenty-five years (Kentucky Nurses Association, 2006).

In 1956, a field public health nurse was appointed to implement a health program for the area. She helped with clinics, made home visits, and taught home sanitation and hygiene. Red Bird Hospital was the only hospital in a 900-square-mile area, and by the 1950s, it needed major repairs. In 1959, a larger hospital was built seven miles away but closed in 1986 due to financial reasons. In place of the hospital, the Red Bird Medical Clinic was established to provide healthcare for the community residents, and it continues that care today (Schaeffer, 1980; Weinert, 1959).

White Rock/Laurel, North Carolina

The establishment of White Rock Hospital and professional healthcare in Madison County, North Carolina, can be attributed to Frances

Goodrich, a Presbyterian missionary and teacher from Ohio. Goodrich made a visit to White Rock, North Carolina, in 1890 after she became interested in home mission work through her father's church in Ohio. While in White Rock, Goodrich immediately saw a need for social service and better education in the community. She believed she could do something about this problem and officially moved to White Rock in 1892. When Goodrich arrived, she commenced working on her home mission project. Over a period of fifteen years, Goodrich garnered support and funds through her father's church in Ohio and other Presbyterian churches throughout the East while she built trust and gained respect in the White Rock community. During those years, Goodrich had also recognized that there was a need for improved healthcare in the community. Once her educational goals had finally been met, Goodrich next focused her efforts on bringing professional healthcare to White Rock, with the aid of the Presbyterian Church Board of Home Missions.

At this time, the only "doctor" in White Rock was Granny Banks, a self-professed mountain doctor/folk healer with no formal medical education or training. Otherwise, the families provided their own form of healing. In a 1912 letter to the Women's Board of Home Missions of the Presbyterian Church, Goodrich noted that Madison County originally had two female doctors: Dr. Helen Bissell, who apparently arrived in 1910 and stayed two years, and Dr. Margaret Whiteside, who arrived in 1912 but left sometime early in 1914 (Goodrich, 1912). There are no records to validate their presence or work in Madison County; however, Goodrich did mention that Granny Banks, the local "mountain doctor," had resented the new female doctor.

White Rock was in need of a professionally trained doctor, and, toward the end of 1914, a friend of Goodrich suggested she contact Dr. George Packard in Boston, Massachusetts, who had compassion for those in need and a strong interest in missionary work. He and his wife visited White Rock in 1914 and, through the Presbyterian Church Board of Home Missions, moved to North Carolina six months later and set up practice in the White Rock/Laurel community. However, as a newcomer in a community suspicious of outsiders, the new doctor faced the significant challenge of establishing confidence and trust among the residents. Packard was considered another "furriner" and "fotched-on" doctor. He persisted, however, and eventually was accepted into the community after saving a local leader's life by performing an emergency appendectomy on a kitchen table, with the community residents

III. Early Nursing Practice

looking on through the cabin window. The community leader whose life was saved was impressed with Packard's care and later sold five acres of land to the Presbyterian Church so that a hospital could be built to care for the community residents. In its 1919 annual report, the Presbyterian Church Board of Home Missions announced that a new hospital would be ready for occupancy that year and would serve as a model mountain station. Dr. Packard began with three nurses: Miss Mabel Rich (a Red Cross public health nurse), Miss Harrington, and Miss Gardner, all of whom frequently worked without remuneration or concern about those volunteered hours (Bellamy 1921; Board of Home Missions, 1919). As a Red Cross nurse, Rich had a strong background in World War I with the Red Cross, in addition to her work as a public health nurse.

In a 1922 report to the Presbyterian Church Board of Home Missions, Goodrich described several days from the work of the doctor and his three nurses:

> Four A.M. Sunday morning: dark and bitter chill. Doctor and nurse leave the hospital on horseback for a confinement case on the Cook Farm Road.... Just before daybreak comes the second call: a woman in labor on Spillcorn, ten miles in the opposite direction. A second nurse starts out with buggy and mules, and with obstetrical supplies, to meet the doctor.... The first nurse, meanwhile, finishing her work for mother and child on the Cook Farm, returns to the hospital leading the other horse.... On Monday ... the first nurse put in a full day, riding twenty miles or more to care for the two new babies and to teach the mothers how to look after them. The second nurse, besides hospital duty, rode in the afternoon to see a patient in need of nurse's care.
> On Tuesday, the first nurse went by the short cut over the Sapling Mountain to attend to the Spillcorn baby and its mother, and after making them comfortable she took the Bend of Laurel trail.... The trail leads ... down the hill, into and up the rushing stream ... then across to the other side by a rough ford and up over the rocks to the height above. Eventually it leads to Revere where the nurse meets with the doctor who has ridden over for his weekly clinic. Before reaching there she makes several calls where her services are needed, then assists at the clinic. On the way home she is needed to assist in three surgical dressings. Twenty-five miles in the saddle for the day's work.
> The second nurse visited the other mother and baby and also stopped to see a patient with heart trouble, to get report.
> Wednesday. The first nurse rode again over Sapling to see the mother and child on Spillcorn Creek, and from there on up the creek to visit a case in the logging camp.... The creek was "over bounds," and the fords hardly safe; in one the horse had to swim the torrent....
> Then in order to meet the doctor, who was ... on the north side of Sugar Loaf, she went over a trail new to her ... not an easy way at any time.... Here she assisted the

Appalachian Nursing

doctor in clinic with several women, and beyond, three miles farther up the creek, in two lumber camps, there were cases where she was needed with the doctor. Home by the Creek Road with a stop at another camp on the way. Her day's trip was thirty miles....

The second nurse had done the follow-up work with the Cook Farm baby and had gone on three miles beyond to do surgical dressings for three badly burned patients who had been discharged from the hospital but were still needing care. In the morning she had been out also, with the doctor, and had assisted with two other patients at the extremes of life, one, a very old, infirm woman, and one, a little child....

> Yours sincerely,
>
> Frances L. Goodrich
> (Tweed, 2018)

Goodrich went on to state that the third nurse had stayed at the hospital, taking care of six patients and office calls. The three nurses had worked together, taking turns with night duty at the hospital, but they did not closely count their hours.

In 1931, White Rock Hospital fell victim to the Great Depression and went bankrupt. A few nurses stayed on to provide medical service to residents of the community, living in the doctor's hospital manse until sometime during the 1940s (Tabler, 2019).

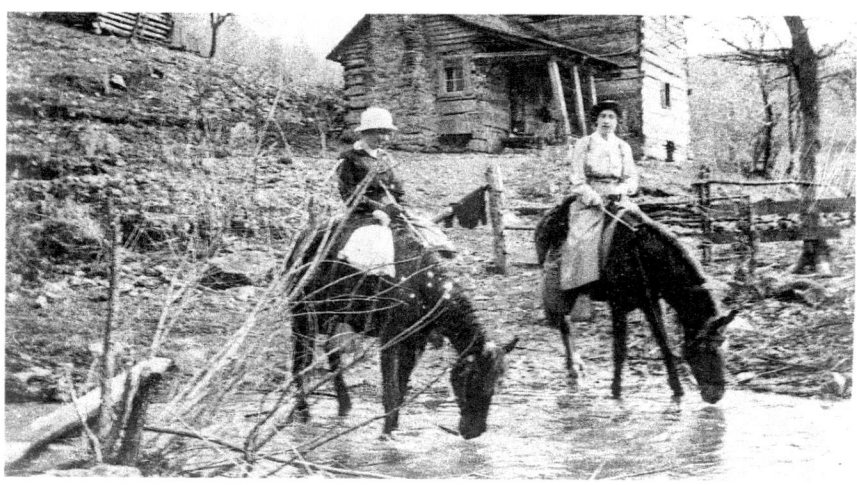

Mabel Rich, RN, Red Cross nurse in the mountains of North Carolina, 1919. Her location in the photo is not specified but she is probably at left (American Red Cross Public Health Nursing).

III. Early Nursing Practice

Vardy, Tennessee

Vardy is a small community, lying between Powell Mountain and Newman's Ridge in Hancock County, Tennessee. During the late nineteenth and early twentieth centuries, the community was composed primarily of a population known as "Melungeons," whose ethnic origin has been speculated to be a mixture of Native American, African, and European background. Disagreement remains, however, over their true ethnic identity and ancestry. To some residents, the label "Melungeon" was also considered a racial slur (Claude Collins, personal communication [interview], June 21, 2015).

During the late 1890s and early 1900s, Vardy was a poor, isolated community where residents faced discrimination and isolation; however, they were self-sufficient and raised what was necessary for food, farmed tobacco, made moonshine, and bartered with their neighbors. In 1892, the Presbyterian Church Board of Home Missions in New York City established a mission in Vardy to address the socioeconomic and educational issues that plagued the community. It began with the foundation of a small church and then expanded into a school that became central to the community as a source of education and healthcare for the local residents. In 1910, Mary Rankin (born in Scotland, raised and educated in Minnesota) arrived in Vardy as a missionary and teacher. Her primary role was to teach the residents' children in the community school. In addition to teaching, Rankin was a "Bible Reader," and, on Sundays, she taught Sunday school to the students and their parents. Rankin did not have a background in nursing; however, Vardy was an isolated community, and the nearest physician was over twenty miles away, so, in the absence of a locally available medical professional, Rankin also became the community nurse, providing much-needed basic healthcare for the residents. She was well respected in the community, and although she had never received professional nurses' training, Vardy residents referred to Rankin as their "nurse."

Rankin had a degree in education from Macalester College in Minnesota. She read medical journals, was resourceful, and kept in touch with her family doctor in Minnesota, contacting him when she encountered a health problem that she did not know how to treat or had questions. The doctor provided her with step-by-step instructions on how to handle medical and health-related problems when she needed guidance. From 1920 to 1921, Rankin took a leave of absence from the Presbyterian

Appalachian Nursing

Home Mission and Vardy to attend Teachers College at Columbia University in New York City, where she received a master's degree in rural education. Courses for this degree included rural health. After her graduation, Rankin returned to Vardy and continued her work in teaching and providing healthcare to residents of the community. She was known to make home visits by mule, instead of using a horse. Many of the cabins were located atop Newman's Ridge and Powell Mountain, and mules were known to have steadier footing for navigating steep mountainous terrain. While Rankin provided healthcare to the community, she was very concerned about malnutrition among children to the extent that she created a milk stop for children whose parents did not have the resources for additional milk. Rankin arranged for those children to stop at specific community members' homes for a glass of milk on the way to school every morning. Rankin also served as a midwife, delivering many Vardy babies, and stated:

> You know, when a woman's having a baby, you can't wait on the doctor to come over the mountain! I was always there at the birthings to help.... I showed the mothers how to take care of themselves and their babies, so they'd all be clean and healthy [Frady, 1974, p. I-E].

Rankin became actively involved in the treatment of hookworm and care of the children in the community. Hookworm, spread through contaminated soil, was a prevalent disease in the region during the late nineteenth to mid-twentieth centuries, particularly among children because they frequently went barefoot. Vardy, being a very rural, small community in the core Appalachian region, was not spared. Rankin followed medical guidelines and, in an interview years later, described her experience with hookworm:

> Well... when I got there, everybody had hookworms and roundworms. The children were weak with it. I sent for some medicine and told them if they took it, they would be cured. When it arrived, I had to show them the medicine wouldn't hurt them, so I swallowed the first spoonful while they watched. Most of the children wouldn't take it at home. They'd come to my house, and I gave it. I'd put a little sugar with it to make it go down a little easier. And when it started working, people came from other valleys to take the cure so I had to get more medicine ... and I did! ... they trusted me [Frady, 1974, p. I-E].

Eventually, Rankin was successful in eradicating hookworm among the children in Vardy. In a 1930 *Journal of the American Medical Association* article, Dr. G.F. Otto mentioned the Vardy community and its

III. Early Nursing Practice

favorable results in reducing the incidence of hookworm (Frady, 1974; Otto, 1930).

Pi Beta Phi, Gatlinburg, Tennessee

Pi Beta Phi is a fraternity for women with a strong focus on literacy and altruism; it was founded in 1867 at Monmouth College, Monmouth, Illinois, and is still in existence today. In 1910, the fraternity decided to create a national service project and searched for a community in need of educational outreach. Gatlinburg, Tennessee, was selected. Unlike other settlement schools in the Appalachian region that were sponsored by religious organizations, the Pi Beta Phi Settlement School was established without any affiliation to any church or religious organization.

In addition to the isolation and poverty of the families in the community, the school administrators recognized that there was a serious lack of healthcare for community residents and took steps to address this problem.

In the fall of 1920, Canadian-born Phyllis Higinbotham, a 1918 graduate of the Johns Hopkins nurses' training program with a master's degree from Columbia University, experience in New York City settlement work, and a military nursing background during World War I, was hired as the first Pi Beta Phi Settlement School nurse. She began her work without an office or supplies, but eventually an old cottage in the community was donated to the school and converted into a small hospital. It was dedicated in May 1922 as the Jennie Nicholl Memorial Hospital (in honor of a pioneer doctor in the community, Jennie Nicholl) and provided Higinbotham with space to work. For six years following her arrival at the settlement school, Higinbotham continued to provide nursing services and make home visits to residents in the community. In addition, she taught hygiene and a class for midwives. Doctors helped expand her medical knowledge while continuing to provide her with support and aid; in timer, the small hospital became known as a model rural health center. After visiting the center, a prominent doctor from Memphis wrote a report advising the state of Tennessee to use that center as a model for rural health centers throughout the state (Higinbotham, 1923).

In 1921, Higinbotham described one of her experiences making a 10-mile trip to the "Sugar Lands" on her horse "Dan" to visit a family whose child was sick, followed by notes regarding her work with the schoolchildren:

Appalachian Nursing

> The roads at present are terrible; Dan's feet went "squishy squashy" through the dreadful muddy clay of Mill Creek hill.... Our progress was slow, for the road beside being very rocky was constantly ascending.... Dan, tied to the fence, viewed what he could of the landscape while I went in to see the sick boy.... This last week most of my spare time has been spent over in the school examining the sight and hearing of the children in the primary grades.... It is quite a novelty to them, and, far from being afraid, they usually say "my turn next"[;] a classroom examination of eyes and mouths showed 79% needing attention of some kind [Higgenbothan (sic), 1921, pp. 335–337].

Higinbotham wrote an article titled "Nursing in the Mountains" describing her experiences, including a visit six months after her arrival in Tennessee, at which time she met with Mabel Rich, a registered nurse in White Rock, North Carolina. Higinbotham appreciated advice about nursing in the rural Appalachian region that was offered to her by Rich during that visit and came back to Sevier County with her "head above water and ... fresh inspiration." Higinbotham found that nursing and healthcare in a rural and isolated setting was far different from nursing practices in the city, and she set out to prepare herself for the rural setting:

> I have practically three sets of equipment, one for office use, one for my saddle bags and one for the obstetrical bag which I found necessary to acquire a year ago, as sometimes it is impossible for the people to get to a doctor in time [Higinbotham, 1923, p. 638].

Higinbotham soon learned how community residents in this rural area sometimes delayed seeking assistance for illness:

> Infectious diseases are apt to be severer than one finds in the cities; for instance diphtheria gains fearful headway before any attempt is made to get help and the antitoxin is seldom given early—if at all. As to small pox vaccination, they would much prefer the disease [Higinbotham, 1923, p. 635].

She also described how distance was an important factor in making home visits and noted the importance of keeping her district within a "five-mile radius": "when I have to make calls outside of it one visit will often take all day." During one long day, Higinbotham recounted:

> Coming home after dark one night I found a call to see a baby that the father thought had membranous croup. It was about the farthest place in another community. Taking all the emergency antitoxin I had, one of the teachers drove me as far as possible in a Ford, then we walked through the woods to the house and gave the antitoxin by the help of a smoky lamp and a

III. Early Nursing Practice

flashlight.... The child couldn't have lived till morning so there was no waiting to get a doctor—the nearest one couldn't have been gotten under six or eight hours provided he was at home when called [Higinbotham, 1923, p. 635].

Doctors in nearby Sevierville and Knoxville were impressed with Higinbotham's nursing capabilities and the work she was doing. Higinbotham felt the doctors were not only loyal but also very supportive of her. They stood behind her for everything she had been doing and taught her medical procedures that went beyond nursing. Although she made it a rule not to go in place of a doctor unless one could not be reached, the doctors had provided her with additional education, knowing that they would not always be available for emergencies, and she gave them significant credit for that education:

> [T]here could have been no running without the loyalty, support, and help of the doctors. It was they who, while not living here, came into the district when called, who paved the way for a nurse, have stood firm and strong for everything done and have taught me much that belongs to the sphere of a doctor because they felt there would be emergencies to be met when they weren't here [Higinbotham, 1923, p. 638].

Higinbotham concluded:

> Nursing in the mountains may sound like nothing but problems and difficulties but the compensation more than makes up for them. First, the people themselves are wonderful to work with and for; so are the doctors ... the longer one stays the more fascinating the work becomes [Higinbotham, 1923, p. 638].

After Higinbotham resigned, a number of nurses practiced at the Pi Beta Phi settlement health center, including Frances Moore, a school nurse and graduate of Cook County Hospital and the University of Chicago. Moore left Pi Beta Phi after three years to teach at East Tennessee State Teacher's College in Johnson City, Tennessee. In 1936, Marjorie Chalmers, a graduate of the nurses' training program at Eitel Hospital in Minneapolis, Minnesota, was hired as a "School and Community Nurse" for Pi Beta Phi; she planned to stay for approximately a year. In her memoir about the experiences at Pi Beta Phi, Chalmers recalled her first perceptions of the region when she arrived and her lack of preparation for what she was about to encounter:

> How did I let myself get talked into taking this position? I knew nothing about Public Health, I never heard of the Pi Beta Phi Settlement School.

Appalachian Nursing

> I couldn't even find Gatlinburg on my map of Tennessee. My experiences with mountain roads was confined to glimpses from a train window. I hadn't ridden a horse for years.... I felt my qualifications for a mountain nurse rated low [Chalmers, 1975, p. 7].

The nurse whom Chalmers replaced stayed with her for less than a week, and then Chalmers was on her own. She enjoyed the beauty of the mountains and shared how she navigated the geography:

> I learned to drive slowly and smoothly when there was no place to go but in the stream bed itself—fording the creek lengthwise saves cutting off the banks for a road and saves scarce flat land.... I had learned long since to leave my clothes in order as a fireman does, and prided myself on my ability to be ready for the road less than ten minutes after a call had come in. I learned to sterilize instruments in a basin propped over red coals on the hearth, to improvise a croup tent with a light blanket and an umbrella, sitting under the tent with a child in my arms [Chalmers, 1975, p. 20].

Chalmers remained at Pi Beta Phi for more than the originally planned one year, retiring 27 years later in 1962 (Gordon, 1962).

Industrialization, the Railroad, and Coal Mining

With the industrialization of Appalachia, the railroad, coal mining, and lumber emerged as flourishing industries in the region. Toward the mid- to latter part of the nineteenth century, the core of Appalachia had experienced extraordinary industrial growth in rail, coal, and lumber. As a result, a flood of workers and their families began moving into the region from across the United States.

Railroad companies were expanding their lines into the less populated areas of the Appalachian region. Coal mining companies in northern Appalachia began to establish company towns in the core region. The industrial boom of rail and coal industries had significantly expanded in the area; however, in addition to new workers and their families, this new growth brought with it occupational risks.

New towns emerged and existing ones grew with the expansion of these industries. The growing population in the core of Appalachia gave rise to an increase in accidents, injuries, and illness associated with not only the coal and railroad industries but also timber. The need for hospitals, doctors, and nurses to take care of the workers and their families

III. Early Nursing Practice

likewise grew. Access to healthcare, professionally educated physicians, and hospitals in the region was limited. Soon there were not enough professionally educated physicians to care for the growing population of workers suffering from industrial accidents. In addition to the urgent need for more physicians, hospitals located in areas convenient for the workers became essential in order to provide care following industrial accidents, injuries, or illness. Another issue that complicated access to professional healthcare was that among most community residents, there was distrust of doctors and nurses who came from outside the region. Local residents were loyal to their traditional healers (Barney, 1996). It took time for providers who were new to the region to establish trust and respect in order to be accepted within the Appalachian communities. Prior to the arrival of professional medicine, most residents had turned to grannies and yarb doctors for treatment, and the professionally educated doctors tended to create competition in the region.

The Railroad Industry and Healthcare

During the mid-nineteenth century, the railroad industry had begun expanding into the Appalachian core region, as it provided a more economical and convenient way to transport coal than bringing it down from the mountains, placing it on barges, and shipping by river waterways. In 1870, there was one railroad in the Southern Appalachian region, but by 1900 there were four. With the growing rail network that extended all the way through to the Kentucky coalfields, the need for additional medical care services in the region became evident due to the serious injuries resulting from rail accidents among the workers. It soon became apparent that there were not enough local hospitals to provide timely care for industrial accidents or illnesses.

In Chattanooga, Tennessee, officials determined that it took too long to transport injured workers to the closest hospital in Knoxville, which was over 100 miles away. Baron Frederic Emile d'Erlanger of France had financial stakes in several railroad companies in the region and, in 1889, made a visit to Chattanooga to check on his interests. He expressed concern about the length of time required to transport an injured railroad worker from Chattanooga to Knoxville. As a result of his observations, d'Erlanger recognized that there was a significant need for quick access to a hospital for railroad workers, and he donated $5,000 toward construction of a hospital in Chattanooga that would take care of rail employees who had been injured in their work. Inspired by d'Erlanger's initial donation, the Chattanooga Hospital Association embarked on a campaign to raise additional funds that were needed to complete the hospital. After a series of financial challenges, the Baroness Erlanger Hospital (named after his wife) opened in 1899. That same year, one of the first professional nurses' training schools in the state of Tennessee was established at Baroness Erlanger Hospital with an inaugural class of five students who graduated two years later in 1901 (Poole & Sawyer, 1993).

During the same period in another part of Southern Appalachia, the Chesapeake and Ohio Railway Employee Hospital Association was established with the purpose of providing workers and their families in Virginia and West Virginia with convenient access to healthcare. Two hospitals were built near the railroad line—one in Clifton Forge, Virginia, and the other in Huntington, West Virginia. Nurses' training schools were also established in each hospital. The railroad workers paid small monthly dues and received prepaid hospital care for themselves and their families. In addition, the workers and their families were able to travel free of charge to the hospital that was located closest to them.

HUNTINGTON, WEST VIRGINIA

As a way to provide healthcare for railroad employees, the C&O Hospital opened in 1900 in a home at 6th and 18th Streets in Huntington, West Virginia. The hospital soon outgrew its initial location due to rising medical demands, and a new four-story hospital with eighty beds was built across the street. The original building was used as an annex and included a ward for African American patients. In 1915, the hospital established a training school for nurses. The school's first director of nursing was Madge Smith. Applicants to the school had to be between the ages of 18 and 35 with a minimum of one year of high school. Students received 36 months of instruction with training in medical, surgical, and gynecological care. The last four months of students' training in pediatrics and obstetrics were spent at Cincinnati General Hospital in Cincinnati, Ohio. Eleanor Koch, RN, was the nurse superintendent at the time the school was included on the 1922 list of nurses' training schools that had met the criteria set forth by the National League of Nursing Education and was accredited by the West Virginia State Board of Nurse Examiners (American Nurses Association, 1922; Bond, 1957; Trowbridge, Gehringer & Clio Admin., 2016).

III. Early Nursing Practice

CLIFTON FORGE, VIRGINIA

The Chesapeake and Ohio Hospital in Clifton Forge, Virginia, was originally established by the C&O Railroad in 1879 at the Gladys Inn. The hospital housed 50 beds and employed a surgeon, five nurses, and a medical intern. A newer hospital was constructed in in 1916 with 90 beds. A training school for nurses was established that same year. By 1922, there were eighteen students and the school met the state board of nursing's requirements for accreditation. Due to the growth in population, by 1930, 50 more hospital beds were added. The hospital training school was fully accredited by the NLNE in 1938, and at that time there were 28 students and one instructor for the program. Pearl Pope was the school director (National League of Nursing Education, 1939; National League of Nursing Education Committee, 1919).

Coal Mining, Coal Company Towns, and Hospitals

Along with the railroad industry in Southern Appalachia, coal mining provided a lucrative source of employment that attracted workers from all over the United States. By the late nineteenth century, coal company towns dotted the geography of many states in the core of Appalachia, primarily Virginia, West Virginia, and Kentucky. As was the case for railroad workers, there was a significant need for healthcare and hospitals in the region to serve the coal workers and their families. Although injuries were common among both railroad and coal workers, typhoid (caused by poor sanitation in the coal town tunnels, camps, and housing) and black lung disease (caused by coal dust in the tunnels) were additional health concerns in the coal mining communities.

While railroad workers were frequently provided with housing, coal companies created company towns where they provided not only company-owned housing for their workers but also stores, recreational facilities, and sometimes, in larger coal towns, a church, school, and doctor. Healthcare for the mine workers and their families was a significant need, which became an issue given the absence of local doctors or local access to a hospital. In order to take care of the mine workers and their families, the coal company owners had to hire professionally educated doctors from outside the region; as a result, the workers had a small portion of their paycheck deducted for medical care. Otherwise,

Appalachian Nursing

the community residents relied on indigenous healers, midwives, "granny doctors," or family members to provide medical care. The community residents were especially loyal to their local traditional healers, and there was an underlying distrust of any newcomers who came from outside the region, even professionally trained medical professionals (Barney, 1996). In addition, there was resentment among the coal miners who had to give up a portion of their paycheck for company-provided medical care. As these coal company towns grew, it soon became necessary to establish hospitals convenient to the communities that would take care of the mine workers and their families free of charge.

Henry Hatfield (a member of the famous Hatfield family known for feuding with their neighbors, the McCoys) was born in 1875 and earned his first medical degree at the University of Louisville, Kentucky, in 1894. In 1895, Hatfield became the commissioner of health for Mingo County in West Virginia, serving from 1895 to 1900. He also served as surgeon for the Norfolk and Western Railroad from 1895 to 1913 and as surgeon in chief of Miners' Hospital #1 from 1899 to 1913. Hatfield practiced as a railroad and coal camp medical provider and company doctor. As a company doctor in the coalfields, he performed surgeries on kitchen tables, delivered babies in what were referred to as "dirty beds," and cared for workers with injuries from mine accidents. In case of an emergency in which someone required hospitalization, Hatfield had to send them to the nearest facility, which was two hundred miles away; in many cases, the patients died before they reached emergency care. Hatfield appealed to the coal company owners/operators to establish local hospitals where workers could receive emergency care, but his request went unheeded. He persevered, however, and focused on the West Virginia state legislature, where, in 1899, an act to establish three hospitals strategically located across the state was passed, thus allowing the healthcare needs of coal workers in West Virginia to be met. The hospitals were originally named Miners' Hospital #1, #2 and #3. Miners' Hospital #1 was built in Welch, West Virginia; Hospital #2 was located in the New River Coal Field, McKendree, West Virginia; and Hospital #3 served the northern coalfields in Fairmont, West Virginia.

- Miners' Hospital #1 (Welch), opened in 1902; a training school for nurses opened in 1914. The school originally had one doctor, two nurses, two orderlies, a night foreman, an electrician, and ambulance driver. Dr. Henry Hatfield was the chief hospital

III. Early Nursing Practice

physician and surgeon for thirteen years. The training school for nurses closed in 1944 (Bond, 1957; Frazier, 1992).
- Miners' Hospital #2 (McKendree), opened in 1901. In 1910, when the nurses' training school was established, a second building was added to the hospital to house the school. The training school closed in 1941 (Bond, 1957, pp. 1–57).
- Miners' Hospital #3 (Fairmont), West Virginia, opened in 1901. The nurses' training school opened in 1902. The training school offered a two-year curriculum until 1914/1915, when it changed to three years. The school closed in 1947 (Bond, 1957).

All three training schools earned both 1922 and 1938 West Virginia State Board of Nurses accreditation. At the McKendree (Miners' Hospital #2) nurses' training school, students were required to complete two months of probation before being admitted to the two-year program. They had to be of high moral character, in good health, and intelligent with a "good basic education." Students were provided with $10 per month for uniforms, textbooks, and other miscellaneous costs. The students had classes at night and were required to work with patients in the hospital when they were not in class.

In her oral history interview, Mabel Gwinn, a former student and later nurse at McKendree Miners' Hospital #2, shared her experiences as a nursing student in 1921:

> Very often we've had to scrub the bathroom and we had to scrub beds. Bedpans had to be soaked in the bathtub for hours, and then we had to clean those all up, and clean the utility rooms up, and keep those all clean. The doctor was very strict about the cleanliness of the hospital, very strict.... Fact of the matter, I think Dr. Goodman was one of the finest men to train nurses. He really was ... he knew how to handle us, and he knew how to make us work [Nyden, 1981, p. 34].

In his 1992 book, *Miners and Medicine*, Claude Frazier shared memories from his mother, Francis Toney Frazier, a 1915 graduate of McKendree Training School for Nurses. Frazier's mother recalled that as a student, she worked twelve hours a day and attended classes at night. She recalled how the hospital beds were always occupied with patients who had severe injuries and required amputations as well as patients whose bones had to be set and whose wounds needed closing. She also spoke about poor sanitation in the coal camps and mines, where typhoid fever was common. Tuberculosis was also a problem in

Appalachian Nursing

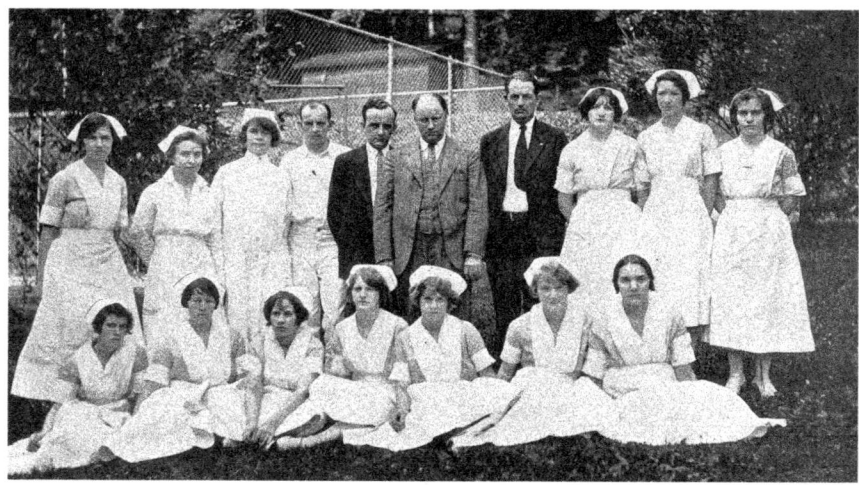

McKendree Miners' Hospital #2—doctors, nurses and student nurses, 1927 (West Virginia and Regional History Center, West Virginia University Libraries).

all three of the miners' hospitals. Nurses commonly administered aspirin for pain and fever, fed the patients, kept them hydrated, and frequently spent additional time on those who needed to improve their strength (Frazier, 1992). Frazier's mother described her experiences making visits in the coalfields as a nurse and wife of the only doctor in the area:

> I helped deliver babies. I took fish bones out of tonsils; I even delivered a baby once when my husband was out on another call. I helped my husband on night calls over cliffs and in shrubbery where there were bears and snakes around [Frazier, 1992, pp. 100–101].

In a 1987 letter to Frazier, another nurse, Pauline Fisher, recounted her experiences as a nurse in the hospital:

> You could hear ambulances rolling in with mining emergency cases and regardless of who you were working for, doctors would step out into the hall and call out. "A little help here!" ... They didn't even say "please." No time for that. And all available nurses would run to help. This was normal procedure for any day [Frazier, 1992, p. 99].

Fisher went on to describe her memories of making home visits to patients in the area and delivering babies:

III. Early Nursing Practice

I delivered more babies at home for ten years than in all three [miners'] hospitals put together.... I would go on location, set up for delivery and manage the labor down until the pains were five minutes apart and call Doctor for help [Frazier, 1992, p. 99].

Well into the mid-twentieth century, coal company towns were numerous and spread widely across the region. Eva Ruth McKean, a former nurse at the Consolidated Coal Company mine in McDowell County, West Virginia, shared her experiences as a nurse in the coalfields during the 1930s. McKean's work involved assisting two doctors in their clinics, keeping supplies in stock for surgeries, providing health lectures in the camp's school, teaching first aid, and assessing school children for health issues. There was a clinic for immunizations, prenatal care and a well-baby clinic. McKean visited the pregnant women once a month and made sure they had the necessary materials for home delivery. Infants were checked at the well-baby clinic when they were a month old and then every month until the doctors were assured the children were progressing satisfactorily. The immunization clinic focused on immunizations for children, as well as typhoid, smallpox and diphtheria for those new to the community. McKean also joined the doctors on tours of the coal camp, focusing on the yards and areas of each home, checking back and advising the families. She recalled that one of the most rewarding aspects of her career was when a doctor from a small coal company requested her assistance for a month to follow patients with typhoid in his camp. An immunization clinic was held, at which typhoid injections were offered. In addition, McKean trained family members in caring for the patients and provided a diet to follow and record. The families followed her instructions, and by the end of the month, the patients had recovered (Bond, 1957; Frazier, 1992).

Stonega Coke and Coal Company was a large coal company town established near Appalachia, Virginia. There were nine camps in the area, and each camp had a hospital, a doctor, and a nurse to provide healthcare for the miners and their families. The doctor and nurse took care of basic health issues, conducted examinations, addressed illnesses that also included childhood diseases, dealt with orthopedic problems, and performed minor surgeries (Torok, 2004). By 1955, the United Mine Workers had built ten hospitals to care for miners across eastern Kentucky and southwestern Virginia. Included was the Miners Memorial Hospital in Harlan, Kentucky, was a school or nursing (Mulcahy, 1993).

Military Nursing

Nursing in the American military can be traced back to wars in past centuries, when women without professional nursing education provided supportive care to the ill and injured in war. During the 1850s in Europe, Florence Nightingale and her nurses pioneered a new way to care for wounded soldiers by providing theory-based nursing case to the soldiers who fought during the Crimean War in Turkey. Instead of simple supportive care, Florence Nightingale's environmental theory of proper nutrition, sanitation, and ventilation formed the basis for care the nurses provided to the soldiers in an organized manner. Nightingale kept meticulously detailed records of the care she and her nurses delivered, documenting the progress of patients' improved health and recovery from illness and injuries. This documentation indicated that the nursing care provided by Nightingale and her nurses led to a decrease in mortality and improved health among the soldiers.

In the United States, the Civil War offered opportunities for women to support the military in providing comfort and care to the troops on both sides of the conflict. These women (and a few men), sometimes called "nurses," were caregivers without the benefit of formal nursing education. At that time, females were not allowed or eligible to serve in the military. However, the United States Sanitary Commission (USSC) provided an opportunity for women to volunteer their services to care for soldiers fighting in the war. The USSC was a private organization created through federal legislation to provide medical and general welfare assistance to the military during the Civil War. During the war, nurses consistently demonstrated a sense of duty, determination, resilience, resourcefulness, and innovation. They gave of themselves.

The year 1873 signaled the beginning of professional nurses' training in the United States, when Nightingale-based nurses' training schools were first established in New York, Connecticut, and Massachusetts. These schools were the first to prepare nurses who were capable of providing professional care to patients, including casualties of war. By the time the Spanish-American War broke out in 1898, there was a cadre of formally educated nurses who volunteered their services to provide professional nursing care to the soldiers serving in the war.

In 1901, the Army Nurse Corps was established as a permanent section of the United States Army Medical Department, allowing nurses a formal appointment in the military. Conflict in war brought out the best in nurses across Appalachia. West Virginia was known as one of the states with the highest number of nurses who volunteered to serve, and one of the first to meet quotas (Bond, 1957; Sarnecky, 1999).

Nurses in the Spanish-American War

The Spanish-American War lasted only a short time, but nurses served a vital role in providing professional care to the military through both the Red Cross and the United States Army. Sanitation in the military camps was very poor, to the extent that diseases such as typhoid fever, malaria, and yellow fever were widespread, creating a significant need for nursing care. Congress authorized the employment of nurses by contract in the U.S. Army, and, along with professionally trained Red Cross nurses, a partnership between nursing and the armed forces commenced. In order to qualify for employment, nurses were required to be mentally, morally, and physically fit. They had to be graduates of a two-year nurses' training school with two years of hospital experience; they were also required to provide a letter of recommendation from the superintendent and physician of the training school as well as a certificate of good health from a physician (Kernodle, 1949; Sarnecky, 1999).

There were approximately five thousand nurses' applications, one thousand of which actually met the criteria. Nurses came from across the United States, including the core of Appalachia. Physicians who worked with the nurses during their service were impressed with their resourcefulness, crediting them with saving the lives of patients who would have died without their contributions and care (Sarnecky, 1999). Lena Warner and Harriet Lounsbery were nurses from this region whose service during the Spanish-American War was lauded and well documented.

LENA ANGEVINE WARNER

Lena Angevine Warner was born on May 18, 1869, in Mississippi, though she moved to Memphis during her early childhood. In 1877, she lost her father, mother, and five brothers and sisters during the yellow fever epidemic. Warner herself contracted yellow fever but survived. She subsequently attended a private boarding school in Memphis, and it was there that she learned about nursing and decided to become a nurse. On graduation from her boarding school, Warner entered the Memphis Training School for Nurses, which was established in 1887 and reported to be the first training school for nurses in Tennessee (and the South). The training school was located in the private hospital, Maury-Mitchell Infirmary, owned by Drs. Mitchell and Maury (Bullough & Sentz, 2004; Greenhill, 1994). Warner graduated in 1889, part of the first graduating class. She also was the first nurse to become registered in Tennessee. When the Spanish-American War broke out in 1898, Warner was hired as a contract nurse and assigned to duty at Los Animas Hospital in Havana, Cuba. She was appointed chief nurse in charge of "Camp Lazear" and Columbia Barracks near Havana, where Warner provided nursing care to patients with yellow fever. The care consisted of keeping the patients quiet, providing fluids such as water or lemonade every hour, keeping the patients' skin moist with a light cover, taking vital signs every three hours, measuring urine output and sending specimens to the lab twice a day. Cold saline enemas were administered for fevers over 103°.

One of Warner's patients was Dr. James A. Carroll, a physician and member of the Reed Yellow Fever Board. Carroll told Warner that he had contracted yellow fever through a mosquito bite, which was new information for her. In an article, Warner wrote:

> My first knowledge of the mosquito as a cause of infection was while nursing Dr. Jas. A. Carroll.... While very ill, he informed me that a mosquito bite was the means of his contracting yellow fever. My record of that day bears testimony, "Patient delirious." It was at that time beyond my comprehension that a mosquito could transmit this awful disease [Warner, 1903, p. 192].

The physician recovered. Warner was interested in the research Dr. Carroll and his colleagues had started at Camp Lazear that focused on mosquitoes, immunity, and yellow fever among humans, to the extent that she became actively involved in their studies. Her role was to raise mosquitoes in the lab for use on patients with yellow fever. Although the members of the research team received government recognition for their contributions to the research, Warner never did.

Warner had spent her earlier years in western Tennessee (outside the core of Appalachia) and entered the Spanish-American War from Memphis, but she developed strong ties to Knoxville as a leader during World War I and relocated there as a public health nurse after the end of the war. Warner became the rural health specialist with the Tennessee Agricultural Extension Service at the University of Tennessee, Knoxville, and resided in Knoxville until her death in 1948 (Greenhill, 1994).

III. Early Nursing Practice

Harriet Camp Lounsbery

Harriet Camp Lounsbery graduated from the Homeopathic Hospital of Brooklyn School of Nursing in New York City in 1881, and she moved to West Virginia in 1890. She served in the Spanish-American War as chief nurse at Sternberg Hospital, Chickamauga Park, Georgia. Lounsbery wrote about her experiences during the war:

> It is very amusing to remember how ignorant we all were of Army ways when we first went into camp.... I know it seemed to me a wonderful thing that my country really needed me and I joyfully went, anxious only to help [Lounsbery, 1902, p. 83].

Lounsbery was in charge of 160 nurses at Sternberg Hospital caring for soldiers with a wide variety of injuries and illnesses, including typhoid fever and malaria. She and the nurses made notes that helped to identify the disease, its progress, and the outcome of nursing care on each typhoid patient. In a 1902 article, Lounsbery recalled the careful recordkeeping that was required of her nurses:

> The close attention and elaborate care demanded by modern methods was given just as freely and skillfully to all of these men as if each nurse had only a single private patient to look after. The fever chart will show how carefully the men were nursed [Lounsbery, 1902, p. 82].

In the same article, Lounsbery wrote about the work environment at Sternberg:

> The long working hours, the unaccustomed heat, and the impure water told in time upon the nurses. The first day I arrived in camp one was sent home in the first stages of typhoid fever.... Time and space fail me as I think of all the pleasant, if arduous, work of that autumn—work that seemed so satisfactory, work that was so delightful to us because we realized ... that we were patriotic, that it was a joy to give of our best for our country, that for once she needed women in her extremity as well as men, and that of all her daughters we only were called to serve her.... The memory of those days will ever remain with me. The loyalty of the nurses, their obedience to orders, their patience when reprimanded, their anxiety to do their whole duty, their courtesy, and the friendships I have formed with some of them give me many happy hours in retrospect [Lounsbery, 1902, pp. 82–84].

Nurses in World War I

By 1917, the number of nurses entering the military had grown exponentially. The American Red Cross actively collaborated with the

U.S. Army to establish military hospitals throughout the country and assume responsibility for hospitals overseas. Nurses from across the nation enlisted and served in a variety of capacities and settings that included mobile surgical, base, and evacuation hospitals. Other nurses had assignments on transport ships, hospital trains, specialty and general hospitals across the United States and Europe. Southern Appalachia was well represented throughout the war by nurses who either resided or practiced in each of the Appalachian core states. The largest number of nurses was from West Virginia, followed by Tennessee (Sarnecky, 1999).

Many nurses stood out and were recognized for their contributions and sacrifice. Mabel Rich, originally from Massachusetts, was a Red Cross public health nurse serving with the Red Cross Commission in Kief, Russia, during World War I. She sailed for Europe on the SS *Red Cross* hospital ship (better known as the "Mercy Ship"), which, shortly after the outbreak of World War I, was dispatched to Europe carrying surgeons, nurses, and medical supplies to provide aid to those injured in combat. The ship's passengers disembarked in England, and each group proceeded to their assigned destinations. Rich was assigned to Unit C at the Red Cross hospital in Kief. She served under Lucy Minnegerode at the hospital until Minnegerode left to return to the United States. Rich then became supervisor of that unit. In 1915, Rich and a number of other Red Cross nurses were recommended by the Russian government to receive the Cross of St. Anne for their service. Rich also received the Florence Nightingale Medal for distinguished service during the war (Dock et al., 1922; Minnegerode, 1915; Red Cross Bulletin, 1919, p. 8). On her return to the United States, Rich joined Dr. George Packard at White Rock Hospital, which had been established by the Presbyterian Church Board of Home Missions in Laurel, North Carolina. In addition to her work at the hospital, Rich practiced as a public health nurse in the Laurel community of White Rock (Bellamy, 1921; Red Cross Bulletin, 1919).

GLORY HANCOCK

Madelon Battle "Glory" Hancock, considered one of the World War I's most decorated nurses, was born in Florida in 1881 and moved with her family to Asheville, North Carolina, where she was raised. Her father was a prominent physician in Asheville and reported to be a physician for the Vanderbilt family (Bandel, 2017). As a child, Hancock

III. Early Nursing Practice

became interested in nursing by helping her father with patients. After her high school graduation, she entered the Presbyterian Hospital Training School for Nurses in New York City, graduating in 1905. Hancock subsequently married a British army officer; shortly thereafter, they moved to England. They were still living in England when World War I broke out in 1914, prompting Hancock to join the British Red Cross. She traveled to Belgium to serve in a British field hospital on the front lines near Antwerp, Belgium. When the Allies retreated from Antwerp, Hancock helped transfer patients to Ghent. She was assigned to a hospital in Fermes until it was shelled by the Germans and had to be evacuated. Hancock then worked behind Allied battle lines, caring for soldiers in temporary mobile hospitals called "advanced dressing stations," moving from battlefield to battlefield with the troops.

In 1918, Hancock was working in a base hospital in Flanders, Belgium, when Anna Maxwell, the first superintendent of the Presbyterian Hospital Training School for Nurses, made a visit to the World War I battlefields that included the base hospital in Flanders. Maxwell described her visit to the hospital, where she came across Hancock serving as head nurse of a large ward caring for soldiers with gas gangrene. Maxwell was impressed, commenting on the limited supplies and resources and praising Hancock and the other nurses for their "ingenuity and resourcefulness" in caring for the soldiers while keeping them comfortable and happy as they recovered (Maxwell, 1918).

Hancock frequently wrote letters to her family in North Carolina sharing her experiences and thoughts:

September 10, 1918 Front Belge

My Dearests, I loved hearing all your news but I got such a wave of homesickness.... I am on Night Duty again and alone and we get 39 and 49 in a night all to be washed and their dressings done besides treatment for most of them and by morning, I am a ressutected [sic] corpse, I really never was so tired in my life. We all are. The staff is so small and they keep filling up with wounded.... Four years of this has about finished me in every way, I think everybody feels the same. Worn out mentally and physically. We have lots of German wounded in, such nice mannered boys most of them.... Poor devils they don't want to fight any more than our soldiers do [Letter from Glory Hancock, 1918].

October 7, 1918

This offensive is taking up all our time. I have never seen anything like it since the beginning of the war. Ambulances for miles almost touching each other. A continuous stream. Hundreds come in and are operated on and are sent on every hour.

> I've never seen such wounds and so many deaths. Dying on the stretchers before they can be attended to.... The mud is so impossible. Sometimes the men get stuck waist deep in the mud and it is impossible to get them out ... if they haven't died from exposure in the meantime and then sometimes they are shot to get them out of their misery [Letter from Glory Hancock, 1918, p. 1].

Hancock earned the nickname "Glory" from the Belgian soldiers because of the work she did in the trenches, dressing stations, and field hospitals (Letter from Glory Hancock, 1918). After the war ended, Hancock and her husband divorced. She returned to North Carolina to be with her family (and, most likely, recuperate from the stresses of war). By 1920, Hancock moved to France and was honored by the king of Belgium for her heroism during the war. She died in France in 1930 ("Devoted Nurse," 1930, p. 16).

Grace McBride

Somewhat disheartened by her work as superintendent of Highlands Sanitarium in Chattanooga, Tennessee, Grace McBride (a Bellevue Hospital graduate) experienced a spiritual calling and decided to devote her time to missionary work as a nurse. She wanted to expand her horizons not only geographically but also spiritually and professionally. In 1914, McBride resigned her position of superintendent at Highlands Sanitarium to enter missionary training at the Southern Baptist Convention in Louisville, Kentucky. After completion of her training, in March 1916, McBride was sent to China as a medical missionary and placed in charge of women's care at a hospital in Hwang Hien. During her time in China, World War I continued to expand, and a call came out from the Red Cross for nurses to volunteer for service in the war. McBride accepted the call, and on September 20, 1918, she and a group of doctors and nurses sailed from Hwang Hien, China, for Vladivostok, Russia, arriving on September 24. Five days later, on September 29, McBride and the other members of the medical group boarded a Red Cross sanitary train that constituted a full hospital. It took a month for them to reach Tyumen, and they stayed with the train until the Red Cross Tyumen Hospital opened four days later. On December 3, McBride was assigned to Tyumen Hospital's operating room as night supervisor. She had planned on returning to Hwang Hien once she finished her work in Tyumen. However, ten days after arriving in Tyumen, McBride became ill with typhus. According to her mother, McBride knew her time was short and had told one of the nurses at Tyumen

III. Early Nursing Practice

Hospital, "I am not going to get well and will go soon; I am ready—I am not afraid to die" (Carlisle, 1922, p. 50). Grace McBride died on December 23, 1918, at the age of thirty-three and was buried in Tyumen, Russia. In her memory, the Red Cross donated $4,000 for supplies to Hwang Hien Hospital in China (Carlisle, 1922).

World War II

World War II brought with it a renewed need for nurses to serve in the midst of combat and turmoil. Filling that need were nurses who volunteered because they wanted to serve as well as those who were members of the Army Nurse Corps Reserve reporting for active duty. In addition, the American Red Cross had a longstanding history of commitment and presence during wartime, and the organization again supplied nurses during World War II for both military and civilian needs (Kernodle, 1949; Sarnecky, 1999).

During their wartime service, many nurses kept journals and wrote letters, while others offered their thoughts years later through oral history projects and interviews. Differences and commonalities in each nurse's experiences and perspectives were apparent; however, their dedication and resilience were unmistakable.

RESSA AND GENEVA JENKINS

Ressa Jenkins and her sister, Geneva, were from Sevierville, Tennessee. Both sisters attended and graduated from the Knoxville General Hospital School of Nursing; Ressa graduated in 1927 and Geneva in 1930. After Ressa Jenkins graduated, she remained in Knoxville practicing as a nurse. In addition, she registered with the Red Cross and automatically became a first reserve nurse. During 1939–1946, the Red Cross certified those nurses who were qualified to serve in either the Army or the Navy Nurse Corps. It was during late 1940 that Ressa was called up for service by the Army Nurse Corps. Her sister Geneva, who did not want to be separated from her, also registered with the Red Cross and entered the Army Nurse Corps. The two sisters were deployed for nursing service to their first choice, the Philippines, because, according to them, it "sounded interesting!" (Bock Pierre, 1943, p. 2). Both sisters arrived in Manila on December 7, 1941, and began their duties as army nurses. When Bataan fell in April 1942, followed by Corregidor a month later, Ressa was successfully evacuated, but Geneva was captured by the Japanese and became one of the 77 military nurse prisoners of war.

In an extensive 1943 interview with Dorathi Bock Pierre, Ressa Jenkins recounted her experiences serving as a nurse in the Philippines during World War II when Bataan and Corregidor were under assault by the Japanese, including how, as a result of the evacuation, she had to leave her sister behind without knowing whether Geneva was still alive or what had happened to her until the 77 nurse POWS were liberated in 1945. Years later, Geneva Jenkins provided a short oral history in which she described her experiences of being captured and held prisoner during the war.

Ressa Jenkins

Ressa Jenkins vividly remembered her experiences during air raids at Sternberg Hospital in Manila:

> Days and nights during the first days of the war in the Philippines seem to run together in my memory. We were in and out of the hospital so many times all day and night because of the air raids, that if we had had a quiet spell for a few hours it would have stood out as an unusual occasion [Bock Pierre, 1943, p. 4].

> There was never any respite from the raid alarms ... the first thing we did was go through the ward to see that each patient had his gas mask at hand ... then we started with the patients nearest the door ...transferring the boys from the bed to a litter.... The patients were wrapped in blankets and carried out and laid on the ground.... At least half of the men refused to go out and we assisted them under their beds. Some would not be moved at all, and some were in such pain it was cruel to disturb them; those in traction could not be moved.... They got so they did not care if they lived or died, and they told us they "just felt numb." Things like this created a serious psychological problem that increased as time went on ... the problem of continually moving badly wounded men became a nightmare. It seemed they were scarcely in when they had to go out again.... If we were dressing a patient, we finished regardless of a raid [Bock Pierre, 1943, p. 6].

Jenkins recalled significant, never-ending fatigue and the challenges involved in caring for those who were substantially wounded:

> We worked continuously all night at the greatest possible speed. Without one moment's rest, and when I was relieved at 5 o'clock they were still bringing boys into emergency. I was utterly exhausted, my brain was numb with what I had seen. The night had been a long, horrible nightmare—my first introduction to war—and fortunately I could not know it was to become the

III. Early Nursing Practice

regular routine of my life.... It was a ghastly thing we could not harden ourselves to—seeing these young boys, eager and full of life, many of them our friends, brought in torn to ribbons, covered with shrapnel wounds, suffering, but never complaining. No one knows how hard it is for a nurse to be impersonal and not let her sympathy and pity get the best of her. The hardest cases were the amputations, and there were many of them—for next to death they are so final. Many boys died in the Philippines that might have been saved if they could have had proper medical care. The doctors were the finest, and they did magnificent work, but from the first, we were cut off from supplies [Bock Pierre, 1943, p. 25].

Jenkins and 47 American and Filipina nurses were ordered to transfer from Sternberg Hospital to open General Hospital #1 on Bataan. When they arrived at the hospital, Jenkins recalled, "Our hearts sank when we saw our quarters, for they were simply filthy ... these abandoned barracks were littered with ... soiled clothing, soiled bedding ... when we walked across the floor our feet swished through the sand and left tracks" (Bock Pierre, 1943, p. 50). Rosemary Hogan, the senior nurse in charge, assigned each nurse to her specific responsibilities at the hospital: some nurses opened the operating rooms, while others, including Jenkins, were assigned to a ward; as a team, they worked to open and prepare the wards for occupancy. Jenkins remembered that there were 24–26 beds in each ward, which were "filthy, even worse than our rooms" (Bock Pierre, 1943, p. 59). The nurses set about sweeping, dusting, and making the beds with clean sheets.

> This was my first time in a field hospital, and I was continually reminding myself that maybe the sand and dust did not have germs out here where the air was clean. I certainly had to close my eyes and forget the immaculate hospitals I had always been in before. By the third day we felt we had perfected our regular routine—clean ward, jump for foxhole, repeat continually [Bock Pierre, 1943, p. 59].
>
> Whenever we ran for a foxhole we made sure we had our pencils, for we always put a pencil in our mouth during a raid, grasping it firmly between the teeth and breathing through the mouth. This lessens the pressure so the noise and concussion do not break the eardrums, and also keeps one from gritting their teeth hard enough to crack them [Bock Pierre, 1943, pp. 61–62].

On April 29, 1942, Jenkins was successfully evacuated from Corregidor by the military on one of two planes. She shared her personal perspective as a nurse caring for patients with extensive injuries and having to leave her patients behind when she was evacuated. Jenkins described horrific injuries sustained by the soldiers:

At 8 o'clock bombing and shelling started with renewed ferocity ... they shelled us continuously from eight o'clock in the morning to four o'clock in the afternoon. Casualties, more than at any time, came in from all of our batteries. Four of them came into my ward, horribly burned when a shell made a direct hit on a gasoline drum. We gave them hypos and painted them with tannic acid and Gentian Violet. I painted one of the men, a Captain, for over an hour, and I was ill from the smell of burned flesh, but the poor fellow died anyway. It was a wearing, harrowing, day [Bock Pierre, 1943, p. 211].

I never get over being surprised at how difficult it is to leave patients I have cared for ... to leave them behind still ill. Makes me feel like a deserter, and I worry about them even when I know they are getting excellent care. I think every nurse feels the same about patients who have been in her care [Bock Pierre, 1943, p. 81].

Geneva Jenkins

To be near her sister Ressa, Geneva Jenkins entered active duty with the Army Nurse Corps in March 1941, and the two sisters were able to work together in the Philippines, although both were frequently transferred to new locations, including Bataan. On April 9, 1942, the army evacuated nurses from Bataan to Corregidor. Due to military policy of evacuating personnel from the same family, Geneva had to board a different plane than her sister, which was evacuating nurses, doctors, and other passengers. This second plane, however, had difficulty becoming airborne and landed in the water, and those onboard escaped to the jungle. Although they tried to hide, the downed passengers were eventually captured by the Japanese on April 29, 1942. In an oral history interview, Geneva Jenkins shared her experiences on Bataan and Corregidor before she and the other nurses were captured:

> The Japanese were coming in so they took us out one night ... and they were blowing up the ammunition dump and they hit our car and we had to get out of the car and start walking ... we just barely made it inside ... the tunnel.... I wasn't there very long ... they evacuated us then ... to get away from the invading Japanese.

Jenkins went on to explain that she, her sister Ressa, and the other nurses stayed and worked in the Malinta tunnel until April 24, when they were again evacuated and flown down to Mindanao on a sea plane. She recounted how she and her sister became separated: "There was a lake down there so we landed there that day and spent the night. The next day we were going to take off."

III. Early Nursing Practice

Jenkins mentioned that her sister had already boarded the first plane and she boarded the second one:

> So we got on the plane. They put another gun on the plane ... they took on more passengers with more luggage.... So when the plane started to take off it went down in the water too low and hit a rock and a leak came in the bottom of the plane. In 5 minutes it submerged in the lake. I had to crawl through the wing to get out of it.... Then we ran around down there to different places to get away from the Japanese coming in.

Jenkins and her fellow evacuees ended up in a civilian hospital located near Cagayan; however, the Japanese found and captured the nurses, took over the hospital, and moved the nurses to other sites and then finally Manila. When asked how the Japanese treated her and the other nurses, Jenkins responded:

> They didn't do anything to me ... the only thing [was that] we didn't have any food.... Some. Very little. Not enough food that we were used to having.... Rice and a few vegetables and at first we had Japanese tea. Later, none.
> We had a library there and I enjoyed reading so I would read when I wasn't working.... Took care of the civilians. The people that were sick in there. Civilians were internees.... They didn't get out of the Philippines when they should have.... I even nursed the commandant one time. He was very sick.... They treated us much better than even the civilians. They respected the nurses.

Jenkins described the day she was liberated:

> The ... tanks came in and rescued us from the Japanese. Liberated us.... We heard these Americans coming. A lot of swearing and cursing so we knew the English. We knew the American [soldiers] were on the way. The Japanese went out to meet them. So they got the Japanese right away [Bowles & Sollinberger, n.d., pp. 14–18].

Ruby Bradley

Colonel Ruby Bradley was born in Spencer, West Virginia, in 1907. She was an elementary school teacher prior to changing her career to nursing. Bradley applied to, was accepted at, and graduated from the Philadelphia Hospital School of Nursing in 1933. The following year, she entered the Civilian Conservation Corps as a civilian nurse at Walter Reed General Hospital. In 1940, she was ordered to the Philippines and assigned to Camp John Hay (Bullough & Sentz, 2004). Bradley was one of the 77 nurses (along with Geneva Jenkins) captured by the

Japanese and finally liberated in 1945. In a 1984 oral history interview, Bradley shared her experiences during the World War II period and her captivity:

> Camp John Hay was really designated as a summer capital of the Philippines.... The climate there was just ideal. It was never too hot or too cold. People came to the high altitude for rest and recuperation. That is the reason we had a small hospital there, just 50 beds or less. People were sent up there to recuperate.... The hospital had only two nurses and one doctor.... We were ... on 24-hour duty, but we worked about 8 hours and then were on call the rest of the time.... Nursing care ... was the same as everywhere.

When asked about the possibility of war, Bradley remarked:

> Really there wasn't too much concern. I think more was going on than we were aware of because my family would write to me and say: "We don't think that you realize what is going on." Of course, we didn't have the daily papers that you have here to get the information. Neither did we have too much in the way of radio.... Then just 2 or 3 days before the bombing of the camp, ... the general unrest, we knew something would likely happen but we thought it could probably be warded off.

The Japanese had been approaching the area, and Bradley recalled her experience:

> I went up about 5:00 or 6:00 o'clock in the morning to autoclave the instruments.... The doctor was called down to headquarters.... As soon as he came back, he sent for me and he said "Don't worry about your gown and gloves..." "We could be hit anytime here..." He sort of half got up in his chair, and ... told me what had happened.... "We could be hit anytime here." ... The planes came over then.... We could actually see the Japanese. We could recognize them as they were looking down at us because they were so close in these little tiny planes. They dropped 56 bombs. It was only a few of them that actually detonated.... The hospital seemed to have a guardian angel because the bombs fell all around it but not on it. The dust was so profuse that we couldn't even go in the hospital to breathe until in the afternoon. It must have been ¼ of an inch thick on all the beds. When the casualties came in, we had everything ready to go ... it was really a hectic day but as I look back over it, it was very well organized because the corpsmen had been trained for what to do.... Our very first casualty was a small child, about a year old. The little boy had his kneecap shattered and he was quite bad off. When he came in, he was really in shock. His lips were blue ... we worked on him a little while ... couldn't get any response so we did a little bit of CPR on him. At that time resuscitation was some mouth breathing[;] we had oxygen, too. It didn't seem to revive him. I said to the doctor "do you think we could put some adrenalin in his heart?" ... He said "Yes, if you want to do it, go ahead

III. Early Nursing Practice

and do it." Well, I got this syringe and I looked at the needle, and I looked at the baby, and I couldn't do it.... I saw this bottle of whiskey in the bottom of the medicine cabinet.... There was some gauze over there and we had some sugar. So I got some sugar and put it in a piece of gauze and put about a teaspoon of whiskey in and put it in the baby's mouth and he sucked it like everything, and it wasn't 5 minutes until he was as pink as a rose and yelling his head off [Miller, 1984, p. 10].

Bradley went on to describe the evacuation and capture:

We had a few days notice that in all possibility we would have to move.... We got out the next morning.... We went on a little path around the mountain that you just put one foot in front of the other ... there were Japanese planes going over us.... When we got to the river to cross it, I didn't think that I was going to make it.... This small Filipino boy ... just grabbed me, bent me in half and carried me across.

The group stopped at a log sawmill camp and stayed for a few days taking care of local patients. Later, on December 28, they were forced to surrender:

We slept the night out on the ground.... It was a matter now of surrender.... The next morning we continued walking down the mountain. When we got there the Japanese were waiting ... everybody was frightened to death.... The Japanese said "There are two Army nurses?" ... They said "You two get off." ... But they were very nice to us. We walked back to Camp John Hay. When we got there we were placed in an old barracks that hadn't been occupied for years.... Our life was cleaning up and fixing up.... The Japanese made some rules. One of them was that if anybody tried to escape, five people would be shot [Miller, 1984, pp. 15–16].

When asked how she was treated by her captors, Bradley responded, "The Japanese treated me very well. They seemed to have a great deal of respect for professional people, the medical people, and the clergy" (Miller, 1984, p. 19).

During their captivity, the medical staff had limited resources. Bradley recalled a patient who needed an appendectomy:

The problem then was how to sterilize the instruments. We didn't have an autoclave to do anything like that. And I didn't want to boil the instruments because the water had a lot of sediment in it. I decided that if we could bake a cake at 350 degrees in 30 minutes, we ought to be able to autoclave the instruments the same way. I placed the uncovered instruments on one of those enamel trays that they had in the operating room. We put them in the oven and heated them.... We did the appendectomy.... He (the patient) came along fine with no infection [Miller, 1984, p. 22].

Bradley and the others were moved to another camp and then, in September 1943, to Santo Thomas, where they joined the other nurses who had been captured. The nurses remained at Santo Thomas until they were liberated in February 1945. When asked what impact the experience had on her, Bradley answered:

> It's made me more tolerant in a way. I don't take things so seriously ... people have never seen their own flag come down and another one go up.... I am more interested now in the political matters of a country—what is happening—and I think nurses should be [Miller, 1984, pp. 32–33].

Ruby Bradley eventually went on to serve her country again, this time during the Korean War.

Korean War

As in previous wars, nurses demonstrated their patriotism, dedication, and resilience during the Korean War. Nurses in the navy usually served on hospital ships; nurses in the air force were on MEDEVAC planes; and nurses in the army served in Mobile Army Surgical Hospital (MASH) units, which were created during the Korean War. MASH units were portable emergency surgical facilities that could provide up to sixty beds per unit. Because of the rapid access to surgery and immediate care in the field, MASH units were found to be effective in terms of reducing combat-related deaths when compared to earlier wars (King & Jatoi, 2005). Although nurses were not allowed to serve in combat, they provided much-needed care for wounded at the battlefield front lines. This care frequently exceeded normal nursing practice, to the point that nurses were suturing wounds, starting blood transfusions, and conducting triage (Tortorice, 2017).

VIRGINIA SNEED DIXON

Virginia Dixon was one of the many nurses from the core of Appalachia who volunteered for service in the army. She was part Cherokee, born in 1919 on the Qualla Boundary of the Eastern Band of Cherokee Indians in Cherokee, North Carolina. Dixon lived there until after she graduated in 1938 from Cherokee High School (a school for Native Americans). After high school, she entered the Knoxville General Hospital School of Nursing and graduated in May 1941. Dixon began working at a small hospital in Bristol, Virginia, while she took and passed her state nursing board exams.

III. Early Nursing Practice

The army had started recruiting nurses, and just after Pearl Harbor was bombed, Dixon responded to a call for nurses to join the military. Shortly after she joined the army, she left to get married. The marriage, however, did not work out, and after a brief period, Dixon decided to reenlist in the army. She was assigned to the hospital at Fort Bragg, North Carolina, when the Korean War broke out, and her hospital unit was ordered to Korea.

In a 2010 oral history interview, Dixon recounted her nursing experience working in several practice settings, including the hospital in Bristol, Walter Reed, and a psychiatric hospital in New York:

> So I got out of nurses' training, and I was working at a little hospital in Bristol, Virginia. And the Army had already been writing to me ... and it was after Pearl Harbor ... I thought, they need nurses, so I wrote my letter and said, "Yes, I'll come," and then they sent me orders and transportation, and I went to Camp Lee, Virginia. And I was there about three or four months, and I went up to Walter Reed [Sanders, 2010, p. 3].

Dixon recalled her experience in the Korean War. Her hospital unit was given orders to go to North Korea to set up a hospital there. Dixon described the building in Pyongyang that they were to use for the hospital, as well as what it was like when patients began arriving.

> [A]nd then we got orders ... my hospital unit got orders to go to Pyongyang. The Americans had pushed back the North Koreans to Pyongyang, North Korea. So we went to Pyongyang, North Korea, and we set up our hospital in this ... it had been a Korean hospital, but they had mutilated it before we got there, like, they had knocked out the windows, and there was no heat, there was no water, it was just a shell, you know? And we set up our hospital unit there, and the nurses ... lived on the second floor of this old building, and we just had cots, you know, little cots, like you'd use in the field, in the military.... We usually folded a blanket for a mattress to sleep on. And we set up our hospital unit there, and we started getting patients from North Korea, farther north ... we got a lot of patients, and they were always in shock because they had to bounce over those rough North Korean roads, and they were bleeding, and we just never got some of them out of shock. And the operating room went 24 hours a day, and you tried to ... you'd do the best you can with what you had, and of course, we all were on K-rations, but luckily ... they would take all the K-rations that came into our hospital unit for all the people that worked there, and for the patients, too, and they would cook the meal.... And it was just bad, because we didn't have heat, was the big thing. We had little tiny stoves ... when you've got patients in shock, you want them warm, but ... it was never warm enough.... But I just felt so bad, because I know that some of these young men could have been

saved if we'd had warm places for them. But when you don't have, you do the best you can [Sanders, 2010, p. 8].

When the Chinese invaded North Korea, Dixon recounted the message that the nurses received telling them they had to leave the hospital: "Get ready, get ready. You have to leave today. The nurses have to leave now, this afternoon. Because the Chinese are coming and we don't want you females to be here" (Sanders, 2010, p. 9). When the nurses arrived at the airport to evacuate, Dixon found that Colonel Ruby Bradley was their commanding nurse. She sat next to Bradley on the plane while bombs were going off around them. Dixon remarked, "Poor Colonel Bradley, who'd gone through Corregidor ... she shouldn't even have been there. Because you're not supposed to send anybody back into an area where they've been captured.... But she was fine" (Sanders, 2010, p. 10). Dixon and the nurses then resumed caring for the wounded in Seoul:

> [W]e always had our helmet near. The helmet is the most useful thing the army had. We cooked in it, we washed in it, and it protected us when we needed.... I remember one morning ... we had no hot water, but I managed to heat a bucket of water on this little stove. And I went around and I poured about that much into each man's helmet.... And I gave this one guy, and he said, "Oh, that's the nicest thing that's happened to me in many a month." He said, "I can shave, because I've got some hot water." And can you imagine, it just made me cry, because here he was, so thankful for six inches of hot water, you know. Just little things like that, I remember. And I wish I could have done more [Sanders, 2010, p. 9].

Cadet Nurse Corps

With the onset of World War II, graduate nurses (some of whom who had already joined the military and were working in hospitals, clinics, and other areas of healthcare throughout the United States) were called to duty while others decided to join them in military service. This situation created a supply-and-demand issue for nursing care in the United States that resulted in a critical shortage of nurses to care for patients on the home front. Not only were nurses needed in the military sector, but they were also needed for civilian service. When graduate nurses were deployed or joined the military, they were assigned to military and associated duties, leaving a void in the nursing care of patients in stateside and civilian hospitals. To alleviate the shortage of

III. Early Nursing Practice

trained nurses, a bill to establish the United States Cadet Nurse Corps program was sponsored by Frances Payne Bolton, a U.S. representative and advocate for nursing education. The bill received unanimous federal approval as the Frances Bolton Act of 1943 (Petry, 1945). The purpose of this act was to accelerate the training of nursing students in order to provide a sufficient number of nurses for military and civilian roles in stateside military, government, and civilian hospitals, healthcare agencies, and industries related to the war (Parran, 1945).

Under the Bolton Act, funds were provided by the government to hospitals with nurses' training schools that had agreed to participate in the program, which was administered by the U.S. Public Health Service and supervised by the Division of Nurse Education. Funds provided to training schools covered the student expenses and also helped expand resources for the schools and their facilities. The program was popular and widely accepted across the United States. There were specific requirements for the training schools as well as the cadet applicants. The nurses' training programs were required to be accredited and affiliated with a hospital. The cadet students had to be accepted into a nurses' training program at an affiliated hospital. Applicants were required to be between the ages of 17 and 35, high school or college graduates, and in good health. Students were provided with room and board, uniforms, and a monthly stipend. They received subsidized tuition, paid expenses, and other fees charged by the school (including books and uniforms). The students also received a monthly stipend: $15 per month in the pre-cadet period of the first nine months; $20 per month for 15 to 21 months (junior cadet period); and $30 per month for the last six months of training (senior cadet period). In addition, students were allowed to select their choice of specialization, from pediatrics to public health. The program reduced the length of nurses' training from 36 to 30 months, and senior nursing students spent their last 6 months in a federal nursing service of their choice: veterans', navy or army hospitals, U.S. public health service hospitals, or the Office of Indian Affairs ("News about Nursing," 1943; Petry, 1943, 1945). The cadet nurse students agreed to serve in civilian or federal governmental services for the duration of the war, as evidenced in the U.S. Cadet Nurse Corps pledge: "As a Cadet Nurse, I pledge to my country my service in essential nursing for the duration of the war" (U.S. Cadet Nurse Corps, n.d.).

The Cadet Nurse Corps program was attractive to students, especially those who did not have adequate financial resources to attend

Appalachian Nursing

nurses' training. Some would never have become nurses had it not been for this program. As of 1945, out of 1,312 nurses' training schools in the United States, 1,125 had participated in the Cadet Nurse Corps program. The core of Appalachia was well represented in the number of nurses' training schools and student nurses who opted to participate. Training schools in the core of Appalachia that took part in the program included the following institutions (also noted are the number of student cadet nurse admissions to their programs from 1943/1944 through 1945/1946):

Kentucky

- Berea Training School for Nurses, Berea (66 cadet student participants)

North Carolina

- Asheville Mission Hospital, Asheville (105 cadet student participants)
- Grace Hospital, Banner Elk (45 cadet student participants)
- Grace Hospital, Morganton (88 cadet student participants)

Tennessee

- Baroness Erlanger Hospital, Chattanooga (432 cadet student participants)
- Appalachian Hospital, Johnson City (61 cadet student participants)
- Fort Sanders Hospital, Knoxville (192 cadet student participants)
- Knoxville General Hospital, Knoxville (181 cadet student participants)
- St. Mary's Hospital, Knoxville (147 cadet student participants)

Virginia

- George Ben Johnston Memorial Hospital, Abingdon (6 cadet student participants)
- Chesapeake and Ohio Hospital, Clifton Forge (152 cadet student participants)
- Radford Community Hospital, Radford (21 cadet student participants)
- Jefferson Hospital, Roanoke (124 cadet student participants)

III. Early Nursing Practice

- Lewis-Gale Hospital, Roanoke (189 cadet student participants)
- Roanoke Hospital, Roanoke (186 cadet student participants)

West Virginia

- Raleigh General Hospital, Beckley (43 cadet student participants)
- Charleston General Hospital, Charleston (257 cadet student participants)
- McMillan Hospital, Charleston (72 cadet student participants)
- St. Francis Hospital, Charleston (119 cadet student participants)
- St. Mary's Hospital, Clarksburg (179 cadet student participants)
- Union Protestant Hospital, Clarksburg (67 cadet student participants)
- Davis Memorial Hospital, Elkins (48 cadet student participants)
- Fairmont General Hospital, Fairmont (107 cadet student participants)
- Huntington Memorial Hospital, Huntington (101 cadet student participants)
- St. Mary's Hospital, Huntington (248 cadet student participants)
- Laird Memorial Hospital, Montgomery (101 cadet student participants)
- Monongalia Hospital, Morgantown (75 cadet student participants) (Robinson, 2009)

Note: While several nurses' training schools in Georgia participated in the Cadet Nurse Corps program, none were located in the state's Appalachian core counties.

Many of the nursing students in the core of Appalachia responded when they saw the nurse cadet recruiting posters. Trudy Fann, Agnes Lowe, and Maggie and Terri Paine were just a few of many dedicated young women from the core of Appalachia who "answered the call."

TRUDY FANN

Trudy Fann, of Cherokee ancestry, grew up on the Qualla Boundary in Cherokee, North Carolina. Following graduation from high school, Fann attended a college for North American Indians in Oklahoma and, after a year, returned to Tennessee, where she decided she wanted to become a nurse:

> I finished that year of college and then I came back to the reservation at Cherokee and worked ... my uncle had a gift shop on the reservation.... I worked for him to get my money to go to nursing school at Knoxville General, old Knoxville General.... And then I went to Knoxville General Hospital and did the three year program and the war started [Simpson, 2015, p. 2].

Fann entered the nursing program at Knoxville General Hospital in 1942. She credited Knoxville General Hospital with giving students excellent hands-on experience (especially learning how to give bed baths) as well as four months in the operating room. During their training program at Knoxville, Fann and several other students decided to "answer the call" and enrolled in the Cadet Nurse Corps. They were given the option of selecting either an army or a navy site, or they could remain in Knoxville for their last six months of training as senior cadets. Fann opted for naval service and, along with several other cadets, was sent to Oak Knoll Naval Hospital in Oakland, California. She and the other cadet nurse students rode a troop train across the United States to Oakland. They lived with 79 other cadet nurses in the Oak Knoll Naval Hospital barracks located at the top of a hill. There were in excess of 6,000 patients at the naval hospital. Most of the patients were wounded officers who had been stationed in Hawaii or the Philippines. Care on the wards was provided by a nurse and several corpsmen. Fann worked on the orthopedic ward for a short time and then on the officers' ward. She recalled that the work was a bit different on the officers' ward than in her first assignment at Oak Knoll. Much of her time on the officers' ward was spent talking to the patients (which she described as "like a psychological thing"), along with giving medications and injections. Fann completed the cadet nurse program, and, after graduating from Knoxville General Hospital in 1945, she worked at Oak Ridge Hospital, Oak Ridge, Tennessee, and later the Mountain Home Veterans Administration Hospital in Johnson City, Tennessee, where she retired 30 years later (Simpson, 2015).

AGNES LOWE

Agnes Lowe grew up on a farm in east Tennessee and decided to become a nurse after watching her older sister care for their ailing father. Following her high school graduation, Lowe enrolled in Fort Sanders Hospital Training School for Nurses in Knoxville, Tennessee. However, she had to delay her entrance until a year later so that she could earn the money to pay for nursing school. Lowe recalled that she

III. Early Nursing Practice

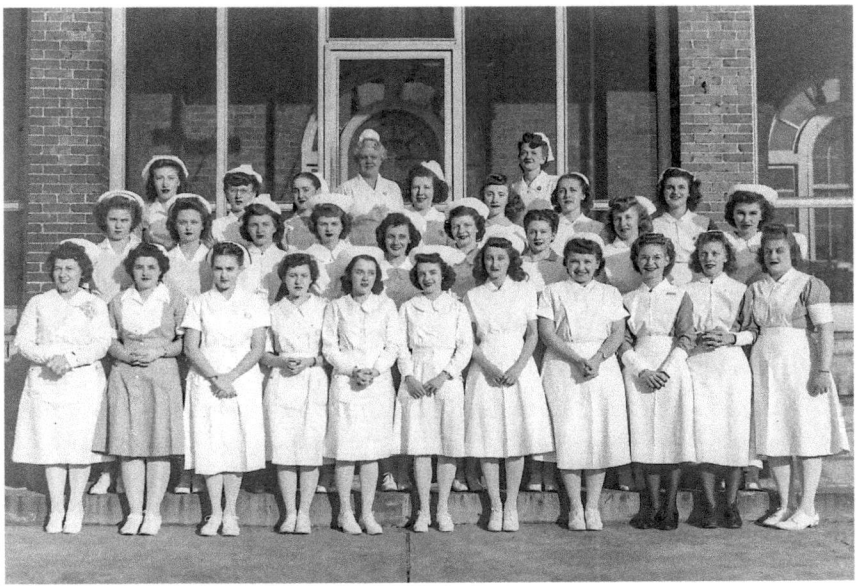

Group of cadet nurses from five different states sent to Mountain Home Veterans Hospital, Johnson City, Tennessee, for their six-month cadet nurse assignment (1947). Agnes Lowe is in the front row, second from left (courtesy Agnes Ratcliff Lowe).

"learned of the Cadet Nurse Corp from newspaper and radio ads" and felt it was "the right thing to do," so she applied and was accepted into the Cadet Nurse Corps. The program was a significant help for Lowe and her family since it offered tuition subsidization, covered expenses, and provided a beginning monthly stipend of $15. During their last six months of training, Lowe and her classmates were offered the option of transferring to army, navy, or veterans' hospitals. Lowe selected the Mountain Home Veterans Hospital in Johnson City, Tennessee. She recalled that other cadet nurse students had come to the Mountain Home Veterans Hospital from a number of states across the nation, including Kentucky, Pennsylvania, Delaware, Virginia, and West Virginia. Lowe reflected on her experiences as a cadet nurse (Lowe, 2009).

> My lasting impression of working as a Senior Cadet Nurse was that I was helping people. This was in 1947 and the War was over in 1945. The fellows were just all glad to be home or back in the USA and not fighting. Some were sad because they had lost a buddy. Most did not really want to discuss their

experiences but we would try to take time to chat with them if they were in a talking mood.... I just tried to care for them in the best way I could. Some patients needed a little more TLC than others....

I am so glad that I was sent to a Veterans Hospital for those 6 months. It was a very good experience and I loved nursing [Lowe, personal communication, July 6, 2021].

Following graduation, Lowe worked mostly in private-duty nursing and practiced at the veterans' hospital. She took time off to raise a family and eventually went back to the veterans' hospital, where she retired 22 years later in 1986 (Lowe, personal communication, July 6, 2021).

Maggie and Terri Paine

Maggie and Terri Paine were two sisters who grew up in a coal mining town in West Virginia. Both girls were excellent students in high school and wanted to go to college; however, their family had limited funds to pay for higher education. Terri worked in the company store to help pay for college, and, with the financial help of a local coal company physician, both Terri and Maggie were able to go to nursing school. Together, in 1943, they enrolled in the nursing program at Charleston General Hospital in West Virginia. At that same time, the Cadet Nurse Corps program was established, which offered both sisters the opportunity to pay for their training. They applied to and were accepted in the Cadet Nurse Corps through Charleston General Hospital. The last six months of their program were spent working at a mental hospital near Pittsburgh, Pennsylvania. Although they did not work in the most violent wards, the Paine sisters did help with patients who required insulin, electric shock, and hydrotherapy. On graduation from Charleston General Hospital, the sisters worked at a number of hospitals across the region until they both retired (Stanton-Smith, 2014).

The Cadet Nurse Corps program officially ended in 1948 (Eberlein, 2019).

Conclusion

Little has been written about nurses in Appalachia, their relationship with physicians, and their contributions to early healthcare in the region. Prior to the mid-twentieth century, there was a paucity of professionally trained doctors in the core of Appalachia, leaving medical care to family members, self-professed "mountain doctors," and granny midwives. The emergence of professionally trained nurses during the late nineteenth century helped fill that void.

While Nightingale-based professional nurse training was first established in the eastern region of the United States in 1873, it wasn't until the late 1890s that nurses' training schools began to emerge in the core of Appalachia. Prior to that time, those aspiring to become nurses in rural Appalachia had limited access to professional training. Some nurses who were trained in the East had a pioneer spirit and were drawn to the Appalachian region. As outsiders, these nurses were initially viewed with suspicion; however, they soon became trusted and respected members of the community.

The presence of nurses eventually grew in the region through the establishment of nurses' training schools during the late nineteenth century; the introduction of visiting nurse services, professional midwifery services, and public health; and connections to nurse leaders on the East Coast. Mary Breckinridge, a registered nurse and Appalachian native, started the Frontier Nursing Service, which is still in existence today.

A collaboration between nurses and physicians also emerged, extending access to healthcare for isolated communities by providing medical services beyond what the doctor was physically able to cover within the region. Working through severe weather and extreme conditions to access their patients, nurses frequently provided care outside of what a nurse would normally deliver in other parts of the country. Beyond the region, Appalachian nurses served their country through

Conclusion

the Red Cross and the military, beginning with the Spanish-American War. Resilient, dedicated, and innovative, these nurses persevered despite challenges and setbacks. The contributions they made to healthcare in Appalachia and beyond have become a legacy to the region.

References

Abercrombie, T.F. (n.d.). *History of public health in Georgia, 1733–1950.* Georgia Department of Public Health.
Alenitsch, D. (2020, December 11). DAR honors homesteader, nurse "Miss Amy." *Crossville Chronicle.* https://www.crossville-chronicle.com/news/lifestyles/dar-honors-homesteader-nurse-miss-amy/article_2d0a34a8-3b23-11eb-aa2f-2f4974524edb.html.
Alvarez, R. (1992). Young nurses long ago: Fairmont's Cook Hospital Training School. *Goldenseal, 18*(4).
American Association of Nurse Anesthetists. (n.d.). *History of AANA.* https://www.aana.com/about-us/aana-archives-library/our-history.
American Nurses Association, Publication Committee. (1922). *A list of schools of nursing accredited by the state boards of nurse examiners.* https://curiosity.lib.harvard.edu/women-working-1800-1930/catalog/45-990091903480203941.
American Society of Superintendents of Training Schools for Nurses. (1905). *Proceedings of the eleventh annual convention.* J.H. First Company.
American Society of Superintendents of Training Schools for Nurses. (1985). *Annual conventions (1893–1899).* Garland Publishing.
Annual report. (1940, Summer). *Quarterly Bulletin of the Frontier Nursing Service, XVI*(1).
Appalachian Hospital and ETSC. (n.d.). Archives of Appalachia, East Tennessee State University.
Appalachian Regional Commission. (n.d.). *About the Appalachian region.* https://www.arc.gov/.
Arthur, J.P. (1914). *Western North Carolina: A history (1730–1913).* Edwards & Broughton Printing Company.
Bandel, J.A. (2017). *North Carolina in the Great War, 1914–1918.* North Carolina Office of Archives and History.
Bankert, M. (1989). *Watchful care: A history of America's nurse anesthetists.* Continuum International Publishing Group.
Barney, S. (1996). Bringing modern medicine to the mountains: Scientific medicine and the transformation of health care in southern West Virginia, 1880–1910. *West Virginia History, 55,* 110–126. https://archive.wvculture.org/history/journal_wvh/wvh55-5.html.
Barney, S.L. (2000). *Authorized to heal: Gender, class, and the transformation of medicine in Appalachia, 1880–1930.* University of North Carolina Press.
Bellamy, F.R. (1921). *The story of White Rock.* Educational Department, Board of Home Missions of the Presbyterian Church in the United States of America.
Bellevue Hospital Training School for Nurses. (1878). *A manual of nursing prepared for the training school for nurses attached to Bellevue Hospital.* G.P. Putnam's Sons.
Bellevue Hospital Training School for Nurses. (1923). *Bellevue Training School for Nurses, 1873–1923: Fiftieth anniversary.* Bellevue Hospital.

References

Bellevue School of Nursing 1889–1989. (1989). *Alumni Association of the Bellevue School of Nursing, Inc.*

Bickley, A.R. (1990). Midwifery in West Virginia. *West Virginia History, 49*(1), 55–68.

Birnbach, N., & Lewenson, S. (1991). *First words: Selected addresses from the National League for Nursing Press, 1894–1933.* National League for Nursing Press.

Board of Home Missions of the Presbyterian Church in the United States of America. (1919). *One hundred seventeenth annual report,* 46. https://babel.hathitrust.org/cgi/pt?id=nyp.33433070799121&view=1up&seq=1&q1=mabel%20rich.

Bock Pierre, D. (1943). *Only a few can tell* [unpublished manuscript]. UCLA Archives.

Boggs, J.P. (1927). Difficulties of remoteness in childbirth. *Quarterly Bulletin of the Kentucky Committee for Mothers and Babies, III*(2), 4. https://exploreuk.uky.edu/catalog/xt7gb56d3d8j.

Bolyard, J.L. (1981). *Medicinal plant and home remedies of Appalachia.* Charles C. Thomas Publisher.

Bond, D.H. (1957). *A half century of nursing in West Virginia, 1907–1957.* West Virginia State Nurses' Association.

Boston Committee. (n.d.). Report of the work of "The Friendly Nurse," Miss Lydia Homan, in the mountains of North Carolina by the Boston Committee, 1914–1952. Papers of Lydia Holman, 1914–1990, A/H747, 4. Schlesinger Library, Radcliffe Institute, Harvard University, Cambridge, Massachusetts. https://id.lib.harvard.edu/ead/sch01769/catalog.

Bowles, J.J., & Sollinberger, K. (n.d.). *Transcription of interview with world war nurse Geneva Jenkins.* MacArthur Museum Archives, Norfolk, Virginia. https://www.macarthurmemorial.org/337/MacArthur-Memorial-Archives-and-Library.

Brainard, A.M. (1922). *The evolution of public health nursing.* W.B. Saunders.

Breckinridge, M. (1923). *Midwifery in the Kentucky mountains: An investigation.* National Library of Medicine. http://resource.nlm.nih.gov/101175890.

Breckinridge, M. (1939, Autumn). Training frontier nurse-midwives. *Quarterly Bulletin of the Frontier Nursing Service, XV*(2), 24. https://exploreuk.uky.edu/catalog/xt78gt5fcm3d.

Breckinridge, M. (1952). *Wide neighborhoods.* Harper & Brothers.

Brennan, A. (1985). *Comparative value of theory and practice in training nurses.* Garland Publishing.

Broughton Hospital History. (2016, April 20). *North Carolina Division of State Operated Healthcare Facilities.* https://www.ncdhhs.gov/media/554/download#:~:text=In%201887%20the%20Scroggs%20Building,%20Melville%20Broughton.

Buck, D. (1940, Spring). The training of frontier nurse-midwives. *Quarterly Bulletin of the Frontier Nursing Service, XV*(4), 18–20. https://exploreuk.uky.edu/catalog/xt7mw6694d92.

Buck, D.F. (1940). The nurses on horseback ride on. *American Journal of Nursing, 40*(9), 993–995. https://doi.org/10.2307/3415250.

Buhler-Wilkerson, K. (2021). *False dawn: The rise and decline of public health nursing.* Rutgers University Press.

Bullough, V.L., Church, O.M., & Stein, A.P. (Eds.). (1988). *American nursing: A biographical dictionary.* Garland Publishing.

Bullough, V.L., & Sentz, L. (Eds.). (2004). *American nursing: A biographical dictionary: Volume 3.* Springer Publishing Company.

Bullough, V.L., Sentz. L., & Stein, A.P. (Eds.). (1992). *American nursing: A biographical dictionary: Volume II.* Garland Publishing

Burke, W. (1846). *The mineral springs of Western Virginia: With remarks on their use, and the diseases to which they are applicable. With an illustration and a map.* Wiley & Putnam.

References

Burr, C.B. (2006, April 1). What improvements have been wrought in the care of the insane by means of training schools? *American Journal of Psychiatry, 173*(10). (Reprinted from *American Journal of Insanity, 50*(2), 214–223 [1893, October 1].) https://doi.org/10.1176/ajp.50.2.214.

Callaway, B.J. (2002). *Hildegard Peplau: Psychiatric nurse of the century.* Springer Publishing Company.

Campbell, A.G. (1984). Mary Breckinridge and the American Committee for Devastated France: The foundations of the Frontier Nursing Service. *Register of the Kentucky Historical Society, 82*(3), 257–276.

Campbell, J.C. (1921). *The southern highlander and his homeland.* Russell Sage Foundation.

Carlisle, R.J. (1922). *A seven years' record of the Society of Alumni of Bellevue Hospital, 1915–1921.* Society of Alumni of Bellevue Hospital.

Carrying On for Jane A. Delano: The Delano Red Cross Nursing Service. (1937). *American Journal of Nursing, 37*(7), 737–740. https://doi.org/10.2307/3413350.

Cavender, A. (2003). *Folk medicine in Southern Appalachia.* University of North Carolina Press.

Cavender, A. (2005). A midwife's commonplace book. *Appalachian Journal, 32*(2), 182–190. http://www.jstor.org/stable/40934393.

Chalmers, M. (1975). *Better I stay.* Crescent Color Printing Company.

Cockerham, A.Z., & Keeling, A.W. (2012). *Rooted in the mountains, reaching to the world: Stories of nursing and midwifery at Kentucky's Frontier School, 1939–1989.* Butler Books.

Columbia University, Teachers College, Adelaide Nutting History of Nursing Collection, University Microfilms International, & Nutting, M.A. (1981). *Adelaide Nutting historical nursing collection.* University Microfilms International.

Comerford, L. (2008, Spring). *Nurse-midwifery in America: European influences on the frontier nursing service* [Capstone, American University]. American University Digital Research Archive. https://dra.american.edu/islandora/object/0708capstones%3A218?solr_nav%5Bid%5D=c6f0dcdb1e93130f69ab&solr_nav%5Bpage%5D=0&solr_nav%5Boffset%5D=0.

Committee for the Study of Nursing Education. (1923). *Nursing and nursing education in the United States.* Macmillan.

Committee on Education of the National League of Nursing Education. (1922). *Standard curriculum for schools of nursing.* Waverly Press.

Cooperation. (1931, Winter). *Quarterly Bulletin of the Frontier Nursing Service, VI*(3), 15–16. https://exploreuk.uky.edu/catalog/xt7sqv3c123s.

Cora Ennis Smith Reeves Commonplace Book [photocopy], 1914–1941. (n.d.). CFMC 454A, Box 7. Anthony P. Cavender Folk Medicine Collection, AppMs-0650. Archives of Appalachia.

Crowe-Carraco, C. (1978). Mary Breckinridge and the Frontier Nursing Service. *Register of the Kentucky Historical Society, 76*(3), 179–191.

Dammann, N. (1982). *A social history of the Frontier Nursing Service.* Social Change Press.

D'Antonio, P. (2010). *American nursing: A history of knowledge, authority, and the meaning of work.* Johns Hopkins University Press.

Davis, C.M. (1917). A bornin'. *American Journal of Nursing, 17*(8), 704–706. https://doi.org/10.2307/3405829.

Delano, J.A. (1933). *American Red Cross textbook on home hygiene and care of the sick* (4th ed.). Blakiston Company.

Delano, J.A., & McIsaac, I. (1917). *American Red Cross textbook on elementary hygiene and home care of the sick.* P. Blakiston's Son & Company.

References

Delano, J.A., & Strong, A.H. (1918). *American Red Cross textbook on home hygiene and care of the sick* (2nd ed.). P. Blakiston's Son & Company.

Dent, H. (2020). *Early nursing department: Home*. Berea College. https://libraryguides.berea.edu/earlynursingdepartment.

Deskins, C.H. (1990). Healing from the hills: Folk medicine of the southern mountains. *Goldenseal, 16*(4), 60–64.

Devoted nurse taken by death. (1930, October 1). *Asheville Citizens Times*, 16. https://www.newspapers.com/article/asheville-citizen-times/35900627/.

Discovery of ether. (1936, October 11). *Knoxville News-Sentinel*. https://www.newspapers.com/image/772700855/?terms=hobson&match=1.

Dock, L.L. (1902). State registration for nurses. *American Journal of Nursing, 2*(12), 979–985. https://doi.org/10.2307/3401951.

Dock, L.L. (1906). The progress of registration. *American Journal of Nursing, 6*(5), 297–305. https://doi.org/10.2307/3403568.

Dock, L.L. (1912). *A history of nursing: From the earliest times to the present day with special reference to the work of the past thirty years* (Vol. 3). G. P. Putnam's Sons.

Dock, L.L., Pickett, S.E., Noyes, C.D., Clement, F.F., Fox, E.G., & Van Meter, A.R. (1922). *History of American Red Cross nursing*. Macmillan.

Dolan, J.A. (1973). *Nursing in society: A historical perspective*. W.B. Saunders.

Dunaway, W.A. (1996). *The first American frontier: Transition to capitalism in Southern Appalachia, 1700–1860*. University of North Carolina Press.

Eberlein, L. (2019). *Making a difference: The U.S. Cadet Nurse Corps*. National Women's History Museum. www.womenshistory.org/articles/making-difference-us-cadet-nurse-corps.

Edwards, P.D. (2008). West Virginia women in World War II: The role of gender, class, and race in shaping wartime volunteer efforts. *West Virginia History: A Journal of Regional Studies, 2*, 27–57. https://www.semanticscholar.org/paper/West-Virginia-Women-in-World-War-II%3A-The-Role-of-in-Edwards/3b6689ef246902db745df4f95ac86a1f3d6c387e.

Ehrenfeld, R.M. (1919). The evolution of public health nursing. *American Journal of Nursing, 20*(1), 14–18. https://doi.org/10.2307/3405424.

Eller, R.D. (1982). *Miners, millhands, and mountaineers: Industrialization of the Appalachian South, 1880–1930*. University of Tennessee Press.

Ellis, J. (1977). *Medicine in Kentucky*. University Press of Kentucky.

Ettinger, L.E. (2006). *Nurse-midwifery: The birth of a new American profession*. Ohio State University Press.

Fee, J. (2002, June 15). *Interview by R.A. Fletcher: Frontier Nursing Service Oral History Project*. Louie B. Nunn Center for Oral History, University of Kentucky Libraries, Lexington.

Fighting trachoma in Kentucky. (1914, April 21). *Bourbon News*, 7. https://www.newspapers.com/paper/the-bourbon-news/1449/.

Flanagan, L. (1976). *One strong voice: The story of the American Nurses Association*. Lowell Press.

Fletcher, A.L. (1963). *Ashe County: A history*. Ashe County Research Association.

Flexner, A. (1910). *The Flexner report on medical education in the United States and Canada*. Science and Health Publications.

For suffering humanity. (1891, July 10). *Philadelphia Inquirer*, 5. https://www.newspapers.com/image/168347339/?terms=paulus&match=1.

Fox, E.G. (1932, December). Twenty years of Red Cross Public Health Nursing. *Red Cross Courier, XII*(6).

Fox, J. (1901, April). The Southern mountaineer. *Scribner's, 29*(4), 387–399; 556–570.

Frady, G. (1974). She went into the hills to do what was needed. *The State* (Columbia, SC).

References

Frazier, C.A. (1992). *Miners and medicine: West Virginia memories.* University of Oklahoma Press.
Frontier Nursing Service Primer. (1932, Summer). *Quarterly Bulletin of the Frontier Nursing Service, VIII*(1), 10–24. https://exploreuk.uky.edu/catalog/xt77sq8qd323.
Gardner, C. (1931). *Clever country: Kentucky mountain trails.* Fleming H. Revell Co.
Gardner, M.S. (1941). *Public health nursing* (3rd ed.). Macmillan.
Getz, L.M. (2009). "A strong man of large human sympathy": Dr. Patrick L. Murphy and the challenges of nineteenth-century asylum psychiatry in North Carolina. *North Carolina Historical Review, 86*(1), 32–58. http://www.jstor.org/stable/23523425.
Gillespie, P.F. (1982). *Foxfire 2.* Anchor Books.
Goan, M.B. (2008). *Mary Breckinridge. The Frontier Nursing Service and rural health in America.* University of North Carolina Press.
Goldmark, J. (1923). *Nursing and nursing education in the United States: Report of the Committee for the Study of Nursing Education.* Macmillan.
Goode, T. (1839). *The invalid's guide to the Virginia hot springs.* P.D. Bernard.
Goodrich, A.W. (1912). A general presentation of the statutory requirements of the different states. *American Journal of Nursing, 12*(12), 1001–1010. https://doi.org/10.2307/3404335.
Goodrich, F. (1912). *Women's Board of Home Missions of the Presbyterian Church in the United States of America (1912).* Goodrich letter (Tweed personal papers).
Gordon, S.W. (1962). News from Little Pigeon. *Arrow of Pi Beta Phi, 79*(2), 26.
Graf, M. (2010). *On the field of mercy.* Prometheus Books.
Gray, C.E. (1918, June). The standard curriculum for schools of nursing. *American Journal of Nursing, 18*(9), 790–794.
Green, E.C. (1978). A modern Appalachian folk healer. *Appalachian Journal, 6*(1), 2–15. http://www.jstor.org/stable/40932250.
Greenhill, E.D. (1994). Lena Angevine Warner: Pioneer public health nurse. *Public Health Nursing, 11*(3), 202–204.
Greenhill, E.D. (1998). *From diploma to doctorate: 100 years of nursing.* University of Tennessee, Memphis.
Greenhill, E.D., & Browning, L. (2006). *A 100 year history of the Tennessee Nurses Association.* Tennessee Nurses Foundation.
Hagley Museum and Library. (n.d.). *History of patent medicine.* https://www.hagley.org/research/digital-exhibits/history-patent-medicine.
Hall, P.B. (2009, November 20). *The Paintsville Hospital.* Johnson County Historical & Genealogical Society. (Reprinted from 1952.) http://sites.rootsweb.com/~kyjchs/painthosp.html.
Hamer, P.M. (Ed.). (1930). *The centennial history of the Tennessee State Medical Association, 1830–1930.* Tennessee State Medical Association.
Hamilton, D. (1989). The cost of caring: The Metropolitan Life Insurance Company's visiting nurse service, 1909–1953. *Bulletin of the History of Medicine, 63*(3), 414–434. http://www.jstor.org/stable/44447620.
Hamilton, N. (2018, December). The evolution of transportation in Appalachia. *VT Intro to Appalachian Studies.* https://medium.com/fall-2018-vt-intro-to-appalachian-studies/the-evolution-of-transportation-in-appalachia-be3f1f738287.
Harbin, R.M. (1923). Nursing as an opportunity. *American Journal of Nursing, 24*(2), 96–97. https://doi.org/10.2307/3407055.
Harbin Clinic (n.d.). *Our history.* https://harbinclinic.com/about-us/#our-history.
Harshman, A.Y.C. (1982). *I remember.* Byron's Graphic Arts.
Hegarty, J., McCarthy, G., O'Sullivan, D., & Lehane, B. (2008). A review of nursing and midwifery education research in the Republic of Ireland. *Nurse Education Today, 28*(6), 720–736.

References

Henry Street Settlement. (n.d.). *Report of the Henry Street Settlement, 1893–1918* (reprint). Henry Street Settlement.

Hess, E.J. (2011). *Lincoln Memorial University and the shaping of Appalachia*. University of Tennessee Press.

Higgenbothan, P. (1921). News from Little Pigeon. In S.P. Rugg (Ed.), *The Arrow of Pi Beta Phi*, 335–337. https://digital.lib.utk.edu/collections/islandora/object/arrow%3A55/datastream/OBJ/view.

Higgenbothan, P. (1923). News from Little Pigeon: Nursing in the mountains. In S.P. Rugg (Ed.), *The Arrow of Pi Beta Phi*, 634–638. https://digital.lib.utk.edu/collections/islandora/object/arrow%3A64/datastream/OBJ/view.

History of the Worth Family in Ashe County, North Carolina. (n.d.). https://www.ancestry.com/mediaui-viewer/tree/151855689/person/372011657uperintent492/media/a462956a-3550-42ed-8758-c4e2ce804ec8?_phsrc=Pny667&_phstart=successSource.

Hodson, J. (1898). *How to become a trained nurse*. William Abbatt.

Holman, L. (1907). Visiting nursing in the mountains of western North Carolina. *American Journal of Nursing, 7*, 831–837. https://archive.org/details/jstor-3402739/page/n45/mode/2up.

Holman, L. (1912a). Our own people. *Visiting Nurse Quarterly of Cleveland, 4*(1), 17–28.

Holman, L. (1912b). Our own people—part II. *Visiting Nurse Quarterly of Cleveland, 4*(2), 28–34.

Holman, L. (1918). *An informal report of the work of "the friendly nurse," Miss Lydia Holman, in the mountains of North Carolina, October, 1916 to October, 1917*. https://curiosity.lib.harvard.edu/women-working-1800-1930/catalog/45-990095179590203941.

Hubbard, R.W. (1950). Public health nursing: 1900–1950. *American Journal of Nursing, 50*(10), 608–611. http://www.jstor.org/stable/3459103.

International Independent Showmen's Museum. (n.d.). *Patent medicine shows in America*. https://showmensmuseum.org/patent-medicine-shows/.

Jackson, S. (2005). *A summer without children: An oral history of Wythe County, Virginia's 1950 polio epidemic*. Town of Wytheville Department of Museums.

Jeannette Paulus, pioneer in city's nursing, dies. (1947, January 4). *Knoxville News-Sentinel*, 1. https://www.newspapers.com/image/772815700/?terms=paulus&match=1.

Jennings, J. (n.d.). Box 57. Joe Jennings Bureau of Indian Affairs Records, AppMs-0051. Archives of Appalachia. https://archives.etsu.edu/repositories/2/resources/419.

Jones, J.M. (1983). *Early coal mining in Pocahontas, Virginia*. Jack M. Jones.

Jones, L.C. (1949). Practitioners of folk medicine. *Bulletin of the History of Medicine, 23*(5), 480–493.

Keeling, A. (2015). Historical perspectives on an expanded role for nursing. *Online Journal of Issues in Nursing, 20*(2).

Keeling, A.W. (2006). *Nursing and the privilege of prescription, 1893–2000*. Ohio State University Press.

Kendrick, J.F. (1939). *Public health in the state and counties of Virginia*. Commonwealth of Virginia Department of Health.

Kentucky Committee for Mothers and Babies. (1925, October). *Kentucky Committee for Mothers and Babies Quarterly Bulletin, I*(2).

Kentucky Committee for Mothers and Babies. (1926, February). *Kentucky Committee for Mothers and Babies Quarterly Bulletin, I*(3).

Kentucky Nurses Association. (2006). *Professional nursing in Kentucky*. Kentucky Nurses Association.

Kernodle, P.B. (1949). *The Red Cross in action*. Harper & Brothers.

References

King, B., & Jatoi, I. (2005, May). The mobile army surgical hospital (MASH): A military and surgical legacy. *Journal of the National Medical Association, 97*(5), 648–656. https://www.ncbi.nlm.nih.gov/pmc/articles/PMC2569328/#:~:text=MASH%20units%20were%20designed%20as,critical%20care%20in%20civilian%20hospitals.

Kirchgessner, J.C. (2000). The miners' hospitals of West Virginia. *Nursing History Review, 8*(1). 157–168.

Kirchgessner, J.C., & Keeling, A.W. (Eds.). (2015). *Nursing rural America: Perspectives from the early 20th century.* Springer Publishing Company.

Kirchgessner, J.C., Keeling, A.W., & Gibson, M.E. (2015). Nurses in schools, coal towns, and migrant camps. In G.M. Fealy, C. Hallett, & S.M. Dietz (Eds.), *Histories of nursing practice* (pp. 180–199). Manchester University Press.

Klug, B.C. (2002). *Twenty-five years of experiences in the Army Nurse Corps (1943–1968).* Vantage Press.

Knowles, S. (2017). Pi Beta Phi Settlement School. *Tennessee Encyclopedia.* http://tennesseeencyclopedia.net/entries/pi-beta-phi-settlement-school/.

Lagemann, E.C. (Ed.). (1983). *Nursing history: New perspectives, new possibilities.* Teachers College Press.

Letter from Glory Hancock. (1918). *Women Veterans Historical Collection Correspondence,* 1. https://gateway.uncg.edu/islandora/search/dc.title%3A%28glory%5C%20hancock%29.

Lewenson, S.B. (1996). *Taking charge: Nursing, suffrage, & feminism in America, 1873–1920.* National League for Nursing Press.

Lewis, R.L. (1998). *Transforming the Appalachian countryside.* University of North Carolina Press.

Lexington Herald. (1919, October 21). *Lexington Herald,* 2.

Lounsbery, H.C. (1902). Some reminiscences of Sternberg Hospital. *American Journal of Nursing, 3*(2), 81–84. http://dx.doi.org/10.2307/3402191.

Mackenzie, Sir L. (1928, September). Dedication address. *Quarterly Bulletin of the Frontier Nursing Service, IV*(2), 3–8.

Mapping Appalachia. (n.d.). *Loosely constructed Appalachia.* https://mapappalachia.geography.vt.edu/about/loosely-constructed-appalachia.

Masters, H.P. (2005). *A study of the Southern Appalachian granny-women related to childbirth prevention measures.* Thesis, East Tennessee State University. https//dc.etsu.edu/etd/1004.

Maxwell, A.C. (1918). What Presbyterian Hospital (New York) nurses are doing. *American Journal of Nursing, 18*(8), 727–728. https://doi.org/10.2307/3405881.

McAllister, J.T. (2017). *Historical sketches of Virginia hot springs, warm sulphur springs, and Bath County, Virginia.* Andesite Press.

McBride, G. (1910). Letter, Grace McBride to Mary Au McBride, October 28, 1910—Enthusiasm for Nursing. https://singlemissionarywwlnurse.omeka.net/exhibits/show/gmnur/item/26.

McBride, G. (1912). Letter, Grace McBride to Mary Au McBride, August 18, 1912—New Position. https://singlemissionarywwlnurse.omeka.net/items/show/30.

McCallister, R. (1999). *Frontier medicine: Practitioners, practices, and remedies on America's first frontier, Northeast Tennessee, 1770–1850.* Rocky Mount Museum Press.

McElree, R.L. (1894). *Home treatment of female diseases.* National Library of Medicine. http://resource.nlm.nih.gov/101562972.

McIsaac, I. (1912). The Army Nurse Corps. *American Journal of Nursing, 13*(3), 172–176.

Metropolitan Life Insurance Company. (1914). *Metropolitan Life Insurance Company: Its history, its present position in the insurance world, its home office building, and its work carried on therein.* Metropolitan Insurance Company.

References

Miller, C.J. (1984). *Army Nurse Corps Oral History Program: Colonel Ruby G. Bradley.* MacArthur Museum Archives, Norfolk, Virginia.

Minnegerode, L. (1915). The Red Cross. *American Journal of Nursing, 16*(3), 220–226. https://doi.org/10.2307/3406336.

Mitchell, S.W. (1894). Address before the fiftieth annual meeting of the American Medico-Psychological Association, held in Philadelphia, May 16th, 1894 [classical article]. *American Journal of Psychiatry, 151*(6 Suppl), 28–36. https://doi.org/10.1176/ajp.151.6.28.

Monahan, E.M., & Neidel-Greenlee, R. (2000). *All this hell: US nurses imprisoned by the Japanese.* University of Kentucky Press.

Montell, W.L. (2015). The Frontier Nursing Service. *Tales from Kentucky Nurses* (pp. 5–28). University Press of Kentucky.

Moorman, J.J. (1817). *The Virginia springs.* Lindsay & Blakiston.

Moorman, J.J. (1859). *The Virginia springs, and springs of the South and West.* J.B. Lippincott & Company.

Mulcahy, R. (1993). Health care in the coal fields: The Miners Memorial Hospital Association. *The Historian, 55*(4), 641–656. http://www.jstor.org/stable/24448789.

Munson, H.W. (1934). *The story of the National League of Nursing Education.* W.B. Saunders.

Murphy, P. (1897). *Biennial Report of the Board of Public Charities of North Carolina, 1897–1898.* North Carolina Board of Public Charities.

Murphy, P.L. (n.d.). Report of the State Hospital at Morganton, North Carolina, from December 1, 1894 to December 1, 1896. (Winston: M.I. and J.C. Stewart., 1897), 9.

National League of Nursing. (2018). *Celebrating 125 years of leadership in nursing education.* https://www.nln.org/docs/default-source/uploadedfiles/about/commemorativebook2018-11-single-page.pdf?sfvrsn=4817a40d_0.

National League of Nursing Education. (1919). *Proceedings of the twenty-fourth annual convention of the National League of Nursing Education.* Williams & Wilkins Company.

National League of Nursing Education. (1922). *Standard curriculum for schools of nursing prepared by the Committee on Education of the National League of Nursing Education (1915–1918).* National Nursing Association.

National League of Nursing Education. (1930). *Proceedings of the thirty-sixth annual convention of the National League of Nursing Education.* National Headquarters.

National League of Nursing Education. (1939). *A list of schools of nursing meeting minimum requirements set by law in the various states.* National League of Nursing Education.

National League of Nursing Education Committee on Education. (1919). *Standard curriculum for schools of nursing.* Waverly Press.

National League of Nursing Education (US), Curriculum Committee. (1937). *A curriculum guide for schools of nursing.* National League of Nursing Education.

National Museum of American History. (n.d.). *McElree's Wine of Cardui.* Smithsonian Institute. https://americanhistory.si.edu/collections/search/object/nmah_716499.

National Organization for Public Health Nursing. (1937). *Manual of public health nursing* (2nd ed.). Macmillan.

National Park Service. (2021, April). *Orlean Puckett.* National Park Service, U.S. Department of the Interior. https://www.nps.gov/people/orlean-puckett.htm.

Nebraska State Journal. (1898, December 23). *Lincoln Nebraska State Journal,* 12. https://newspaperarchive.com/lincoln-nebraska-state-journal-dec-25-1898-p-12/.

New faces welcome patients at St. Mary's Hospital. (1936, February 9). *Knoxville News-Sentinel.* https://www.newspapers.com/image/772712695/?terms=huhn&match=1.

References

News about nursing. (1943). *American Journal of Nursing, 43*(9), 853–869. http://www.jstor.org/stable/3456446.

Nightingale, F. (1859). *Notes on nursing*. Harrison.

Nightingale, F. (1890). Introduction: History of nursing in the homes of the poor. In W. Rathbone (Ed.), *Sketch of the history and progress of district nursing from its commencement in the year 1859 to the present date*. Macmillan.

Nightingale, F., Woolsey, A.H., & Hobson, E.C. (1950). *A century of nursing*. G.P. Putnam's Sons.

1910 Census. Ancestry Online. https://www.ancestry.com/search/collections/7884/.

Norman, E.M. (1999). *We band of angels*. Pocket Books, division of Simon and Schuster.

Noyes, C.D. (1924). The Delano Red Cross nurses. *American Journal of Nursing, 24*(14), 1113–1121. https://doi.org/10.2307/3408794.

Nutting, M.A. (1923). Thirty years of progress in nursing. *American Journal of Nursing, 23*(12), 1027–1035. https://doi.org/10.2307/3407580.

Nutting, M.A., & Dock, L. (1935). *A history of nursing* (4 vols.). G.P. Putnam's Sons.

Nyden, P.J. (1981, Fall). Mabel Gwinn, New River nurse: Interview. *Goldenseal, 7*(3), 34.

Old time Appalachian tradition and superstitions in childbirth. (2017, November 24). *Appalachian Magazine*. http://appalachianmagazine.com/2017/11/24/old-time-appalachian-tradition-superstitions-in-child-birth/.

Orleana Hawks Puckett. (2012). *Virginia Changemakers*. Library of Virginia. https://edu.lva.virginia.gov/changemakers/items/show/224.

Otto, G.F. (1930). Ascaris lumbricoides: Treatment, loss of worms and reinfestation. *Journal of the American Medical Association, 95*(3), 194–196. https://doi.org/10.1001/jama.1930.02720030024007.

Overbay, D. (2005). *Windows on the past: The cultural heritage of Vardy, Hancock County, Tennessee*. Mercer History Press.

Parran, T. (1945, April 18). Medicine and the war. *Journal of American Medical Association, 118*(16), 1374–1376. https://doi.org/10.1001/jama.1942.02830160034014.

Pennick, M.R. (1940). *Makers of nursing history*. Lakeside Publishing Co.

Petry, L. (1943). U.S. Cadet Nurse Corps: Established under the Bolton Act. *American Journal of Nursing, 43*(8), 704–708. https://doi.org/10.2307/3456272.

Petry, L. (1945). The U.S. Cadet Nurse Corps: A summing up. *American Journal of Nursing, 45*(12), 1027–1028. https://doi.org/10.2307/3417010.

Piester, R. (2011). The history of healthcare in the Roanoke Valley: Volumes I & II. *Our Health Magazine*.

Piester, R. (2013). The history of healthcare in the Roanoke Valley: Volume III. *Our Health Magazine*.

Pittard, J. (2016). *A hospital for Ashe County: Four generations of Appalachian community health care*. McFarland.

Platt, S.J., & Ogden, M.L. (1969). *Medical men and institutions of Knox County, Tennessee, 1789–1957*. S.B. Newman Print Co.

Platt, S.J., & Ogden, M.L. (1971). *The Medical Museum at the Knoxville Academy of Medicine*. S.B. Newman Print Co.

Plyler, J.A. (1980). *Public health nursing in North Carolina: Oral histories of earlier years*. Wilson Special Collections Library, University of North Carolina. https://finding-aids.lib.unc.edu/04230/.

Pollitt, P. (2014). *The history of professional nursing in North Carolina, 1902–2002*. Carolina Academic Press.

Pollitt, P.A., & Moore, K.M. (1992). Appalachia health care: The Grace Hospital School of Nursing. *American Presbyterians, 70*(4), 239–246. http://www.jstor.org/stable/23332618.

References

Polly, P.B. (1976). *God, home, and country of the Eastern Kentucky highlands*. Pansy Brown Polly.
Poole, E. (1932). *Nurses on horseback*. Macmillan.
Poole, W.V., & Sawyer, S.S. (1993). *The Baroness Collection: Erlanger Medical Center, 1891–1991*. Erlanger Medical Center.
Powell, W.S. (2006). *Encyclopedia of North Carolina*. University of North Carolina Press.
Prince, P. (1964, February 23). Knoxville's first registered nurse is pride of Wooddale Community. *Knoxville News-Sentinel*, 49.
Pudup, M.B., Billings, D.B., & Waller, A.L. (1995). *Appalachia in the making*. University of North Carolina Press.
Rand, W. (1929). Impressions of a public health nursing service in the Kentucky mountains. *American Journal of Nursing, 29*(5), 527–530. https://doi.org/10.2307/3409828.
Rathbone, W. (Ed.). (1890). *Sketch of the history and progress of district nursing from its commencement in the year 1859 to the present date*. Macmillan.
Ray, W.T., & Desai, S. (2016). The history of the nurse anesthesia profession. *Journal of Clinical Anesthesia, 30*, 51–58. https://doi.org/10.1016/j.jclinane.2015.11.005.
Red Bird Mission. (n.d.). *Our history*. https://rbmission.org/about-us/our-history/.
Red Cross Bulletin. (1919, January 6). *The Red Cross Bulletin, III*(2), 8.
Reid, D.E. (1992). *Saddlebags full of memories*. Doris E. Reid.
Report of the nineteenth annual convention of the National League of Nursing Education. (1913). *American Journal of Nursing, 13*(12), 1001–1005. https://doi.org/10.2307/3404981.
Review of *Income and health in remote rural areas*, by M.B. Willeford. (1933). *American Journal of Nursing, 33*(1), 91–92. https://doi.org/10.2307/3412834.
Rise, G.B., Numbers, R.L., & Leavitt, J.W. (1977). *Medicine without doctors*. Science History Publications.
Robb, L.H. (1985). *Educational standards for nurses with other addresses on nursing subjects* (1907 reprint). Garland Publishing.
Roberts, B., & Roberts, N. (1970). *Where time stood still: A portrait of Appalachia*. Crowell-Collier Press.
Roberts, L.W. (1988). *Up cutshin and down greasy: Folkways of a Kentucky mountain family*. University Press of Kentucky.
Robinson, T.M. (2009). *Your country needs you: Cadets nurses of World War II*. Xlibris.
Rockstroh, E. (1979, December 1). *Interview by D. Deaton: Frontier Nursing Service Oral History Project*. Louie B. Nunn Center for Oral History, University of Kentucky Libraries, Lexington. https://kentuckyoralhistory.org/ark:/16417/xt7dv40jwn36.
Rockstroh, E.C. (1927). Enter: The nurse-midwife. *American Journal of Nursing, 27*(3), 159–164. https://doi.org/10.2307/3409719.
Sanders, L. (2010, November 12). *Oral history interview with Virginia Sneed Dixon*. https://nursinghistory.appstate.edu/sites/default/files/oh-index-files/virginia_sneed_dixon.pdf.
Sarnecky, M.T. (1999). *A history of the U.S. Army Nurse Corps*. University of Pennsylvania Press.
Schaeffer, R. (1980). *The story of Red Bird Mission*. Parthenon Press.
Schrift, M., Cavender, A., & Hoover, S. (2013). Mental illness, institutionalization and oral history in Appalachia: Voices of psychiatric attendants. *Journal of Appalachian Studies, 19*(1/2), 82–107. https://doi.org/10.2307/42635928.
Scott, S. (1982). Grannies, mothers and babies: An examination of traditional Southern Appalachian midwifery. *Central Issues in Anthropology, 4*(2), 17–30. https://doi.org/10.1525/cia.1982.4.2.17.

References

Shambaugh, H.B. (2003, Winter). The Magnolia Nurse: Patty Norton of Morgan County. *Goldenseal*.

Shannon, M.L. (1975). Nurses in American history: Our first four licensure laws. *American Journal of Nursing, 75*(8), 1327–1329. https://doi.org/10.2307/3423611.

Shifflett, C.A. (1991). *Coal towns*. University of Tennessee Press.

Shirey, R.T. (1944). Nursing miners and their families: The Koppers Coal Nursing Service. *American Journal of Nursing, 44*(4), 347–350. https://doi.org/10.2307/3456240.

Short history of military nursing: Resources for Korean War nursing. (n.d.). *University of Wisconsin–Madison Libraries Research Guides*. https://researchguides.library.wisc.edu/c.php?g=860714&p=6167916.

Simpson, L. (2015, August 18). Trudy Fann: Oral history interview.

Sloop, M.T. (1953). *Miracle in the hills*. McGraw-Hill.

Smith, K.C. (2003). *Orlean Puckett: The life of a mountain midwife, 1844–1939*. Parkway Publishers.

Snively, M.A. (1894, July). A nurse's day in a hospital. *Trained Nurse, 13*, 8–12.

Stahl, R. (1989). *A beacon to healthcare, 1911–1988*. Printing Concepts.

Stanton-Smith, A. (2014, Summer). Cadet nurses Maggie and Terrie Payne. *Goldenseal, 40*(2), 26–29.

Stephenson, R.T. (1947). *History of Johnston Memorial Hospital Abingdon, Virginia*. Historical Society of Washington County, Virginia.

Stewart, I.M. (1919). Readjustments in the training school curriculum to meet the new demands in public health nursing. *American Journal of Nursing, 20*(2), 102–109.

Stewart, I.M. (1950). A half-century of nursing education. *American Journal of Nursing, 50*(10), 617–621. http://www.jstor.org/stable/3459106.

Stewart, I.M. (1984). *The education of nurses: Historical foundations and modern trends*. Garland Publishing.

Stoddart, J. (2002). *The story of Hindman Settlement School*. University of Kentucky Press.

Streeter, C. (2011). Theatrical entertainments and kind words: Nursing the insane in Western North Carolina, 1882–1907. *Journal of Psychiatric and Mental Health Nursing, 18*(10), 904–913.

Streeter, C.A. (2012). *Let me see some insane people: Progressive-era development of the State Hospital at Morganton, 1883–1907*. Thesis, Appalachian State University.

Swartz, V. (n.d.). Box 5, Folder 13. Ray Stahl Papers, AppMs-0546. Archives of Appalachia. https://archives.etsu.edu/repositories/2/archival_objects/132571.

Tabler, D. (2019, March 20). Nurses who are glad to serve & who do not count too closely the hours of service. *Appalachian History*. https://www.appalachianhistory.net/2019/03/nurses-who-are-glad-to-serve-who-do-not-count-too-closely-the-hours-of-service.html.

Tannen, S.R. (1995). *Kenneth Killinger: Mountain missionary*. Warwick House.

Tennessee State Board of Nurse Examiners. (1919). Tennessee Department of Public Health Records, 1879–1982.

Torok, G. D (2004). *A guide to historic coal towns of the Big Sandy River Valley*. University of Tennessee Press.

Tortorice, J. (2017, August 30). Nursing and medicine in the Korean War. *CEUfast Blog*. https://ceufast.com/blog/nursing-and-medicine-in-the-korean-war.

Training frontier nurse-midwives. (1939, Autumn). *Quarterly Bulletin of the Frontier Nursing Service, XV*(2), 23–27.

Trowbridge, D.J., Gehringer, J., & Clio Admin. (2016, March 28). *C & O Hospital, 1900–1917*. Clio: Your Guide to History. https://theclio.com/entry/10482.

Tweed, S. (2016, November 29). *Granny Banks*. Appalachian Memory Keepers. https://appalachianmemorykeepers.org/stories/granny-banks-tuesdays-with-tweed/.

References

Tweed, S. (2018, March 27). *Homespun heroine, part 3 of 3. Appalachian Memory Keepers.* https://appalachianmemorykeepers.org/stories/homespun-heroine-part-3/.

U.S., American Red Cross Nurse Files, 1916–1959. (n.d.). Ancestry.com [online database]. Lehi, UT, USA: Operations, Inc., 2013. Original data: Historical Nurse Files, Compiled ca. 1916–ca. 1959. Series number A1 27140, textual materials, 101 boxes. NAID: 649203. Records of the American National Red Cross, 1881–2008. National Archives at College Park. College Park, Maryland. https://www.ancestry.com/search/collections/2365/.

U.S. Cadet Nurse Corps. (n.d.). *Cadet nurse pledge.* https://uscadetnurse.org/node/150#:~:text=I%20will%20hold%20in%20trust,triumph%20of%20life%20over%20deat.

U.S. City Directories, Knoxville, 1927–1936. (n.d.). Ancestry.com.

Vande Brake, K. (2009). *Through the back door.* Mercer University Press.

Wales, M. (1941). *The public health nurse in action.* Macmillan.

Warner, L.A. (1903). Experience of an army nurse in Cuba. *Memphis Medical Monthly, XXIII*(4), 191–196.

Washburn, B.E. (1966). *A history of the North Carolina State Board of Health, 1877–1925.* North Carolina State Board of Health.

Waters, Y. (1909). *Visiting nursing in the United States.* Charities Publication Committee.

Waters, Y. (1912). *Visiting nursing in the United States: Containing a directory of the organizations employing trained visiting nurses, with chapters on the principles, organization and methods of administration of such work* (2nd ed.). Charities Publication Committee.

Watkins, F.C., & Watkins, C.H. (1963). *Yesterday in the hills.* University of Georgia Press.

Webb, B. (1920, October). Roaming through Virginia with the public health nurse. *Public Health Nurse, XII*(10).

Weinert, D.W. (1959). *A history of the Kentucky mountain mission work of the Evangelical United Brethren Church.* Thesis, Western Evangelical Seminary. https://digitalcommons.georgefox.edu/cgi/viewcontent.cgi?article=1015&context=wes_theses.

West Virginia Women's Commission. (1983). *Missing chapters: West Virginia women in history.* West Virginia Women's Commission.

Wharton, M.C. (1972). *Doctor woman of the Cumberlands.* Parthenon Press.

White, J.W. (1895). *The ideal nurse: Directory of trained nurses of Philadelphia, New York, and Brooklyn.* J. Albert Cornell.

White, L. (1909, October). The need of a State Superintendents' Association. *Nurses' Journal of the Pacific Coast,* 459–462.

Wigginton, E. (1973). *Foxfire 2.* Anchor Books.

Williams, H. (1937). *Times Weekly Edition, London.*

Williams, J.A. (2002). *Appalachia: A history.* University of North Carolina Press.

Wilson, S.T. (1914). *The southern mountaineers.* Literature Department, Presbyterian Home Missions.

Winslow, C.E.A. (1932, Summer). Frontier Nursing Service Primer: Foreword. *Quarterly Bulletin of the Frontier Nursing Service, VIII*(1), 10.

Woosley, A.H. (1950). *A century of nursing with hints toward the organization of a training school.* G.P. Putnam's Sons.

Wootton, N.E., & Williams, G. (1955). *A history of the Tennessee State Nurses' Association for the fiftieth anniversary.* Tennessee State Nurses Association.

Wyche, M.L. (1977). *The history of nursing North Carolina* (2nd ed.). University of North Carolina Press. (Original work published 1938.)

References

Yarnell, S.L. (1998). *The Southern Appalachians: A history of the landscape* (Vol. 18). Forest Service, U.S. Department of Agriculture. https://doi.org/10.2737/SRS-GTR-18.

Zeigler, W.G., & Grosscup, B.S. (1883). *The heart of the Alleghanies*. A. Williams & Co.

Journals, Newspapers, Publications, and Archives

American Journal of Nursing
Ancestry.com
Bellevue Training School for Nurses Annual Reports 1886, 1917, 1934, 1940
Charles E. Young Research Library
Goldenseal
Journal of Community Health Nursing
Kentucky Committee for Mothers and Babies
MacArthur Memorial Library and Archives, Norfolk, Virginia
Newspapers.com
Quarterly Bulletin of the Frontier Nursing Service
Quarterly Bulletin of the Kentucky Committee for Mothers and Babies
Tennessee State Library Archives
Trained Nurse and Hospital Review
UCLA University Archives Library, Special Collections
U.S. Army Nurse Corps History (https://www.history.army.mil/books/wwii/72-14/72-14.HTM)
Visiting Nurse Quarterly of Cleveland

Personal Communications

Collins, Claude. June 21, 2015.
Lowe, Agnes. July 6, 2021.
Price-Jones, Evelyn. April 29, 2020.
Reel, Anne B. June 23, 2014.
Whaley, Martha. April 20, 2018.

Index

accreditation 29, 39–40, 49–50, 53–54, 58–59, 67, 145, 147
Alline, Anna 33
Altapass 96–98, 106, 109
American Committee for Devastated France 117, 122
American Nurses Association 30, 32, 42, 47, 58. 67, 71, 73, 101, 144
American Red Cross 3, 49, 91, 94–101, 136, 153, 157
American Society of Superintendents of Training Schools for Nurses 32–35, 79
Andrews Manufacturing Company 19
Anna Alston, Mt. Sinai Training School, New York 19
Appalachian Hall Sanitarium, Asheville 40, 43
Appalachian (previously Memorial) Hospital Training School for Nurses 51, 64, 69, 82
Army Nurse Corps 63, 150, 157, 160
Asafetida 19
Asheville Mission Hospital Training School for Nurses, 50

Barnette Hospital 41, 46
Baroness Erlanger Hospital 49–50, 63, 81, 144, 168
Baroness Erlanger Training School for Nurses 29, 40, 44, 50, 54, 63
Beard, Mary 36, 68
Beckley Hospital, Beckley 41, 45
Bellevue Hospital 58, 77–80, 83, 132, 156
Berea College Training School for Nurses 29, 50, 54, 59–60, 112, 168
Biggs, Dr. Herman 68
Biltmore Hospital, Asheville 40, 43, 51, 54

Bissell, Dr. Helen 134
Bluefield Sanitarium 41
Boggs, Dr. J.P. 124
Bolton Act 167
Boston Instructional District Nursing Association 36
Boston Training School for Nurses (Massachusetts General Hospital) 25
Bradley, Ruby 8, 161–164, 166
Brady, Dr. E.T. 64
Breckinridge, John C. 116
Breckinridge, Mary 109, 115–122, 124–129, 132–133, 173
Brennan, Agnes 77–79
Burgess, Elizabeth 36

C & O Hospital 168
Cadet Nurse Corps Program 166–171
Caffin, Freida 118, 121–122, 124
Capps, Dr. H.C 126
Carroll, Dr. James A 152
Carroll, Dr. Robert 90
Catawba Sanatorium 52, 55
Chalmers, Marjorie 141–142
Charleston General Hospital 29, 41, 45, 50, 56, 67, 169, 172
Chattanooga Medicine Company 19–22
Cherokee Indian 164
Chesapeake & Ohio Hospital 40, 45, 51–55, 144–145, 168
City Hospital, Buckhannon 41, 45
City Hospital, Knoxville 75
City Hospital, Louisville 32
City Hospital, Morgantown 41, 47, 53, 57
Civil War 10, 150
Clarence Barker Memorial Hospital 40, 43, 51, 54
Connecticut Training School for Nurses 25

189

Index

Cook Hospital, Fairmont 41, 44, 46, 66–67
Corbitt, Alma, 56, 67
Core of Appalachia 119, 142, 147, 153, 168
Corregidor 157–160, 166
Cox, Amelia Young 54, 63–64, 82–83, 93
Crandall, Ella 36

Darche, Louise 32
Davis Memorial Hospital 41, 46, 52, 56, 169
Delano Nursing Service 96–97
Dixon, Virginia Sneed 164, 166
Dock, Lavinia 32, 34, 94–95, 154
Dorothea Dix Hospital 87

East Tennessee Hospital for the Insane 87
East Tennessee Medicine Company 19
East Tennessee State College 64, 69–70, 84

Fairmont Hospital (Miners Hospital #3) 41, 46, 67
Fann, Trudy 169–170
Fisher, Pauline 148
Fitzgerald, F. Scott 90
Fitzgerald, Zelda 90
Flexner Report 67
Flower Mission and Associated Charities NC 97–98
Foley, Edna 36
Fort Sanders Hospital 51, 55, 86, 168, 170
Frazier, Claude 147–149
Frazier, Toney 147
Frontier Nursing Service 6, 109, 112, 115, 116–117, 119–120
Fye, Mae 67

Gardner, Mary 36, 135
George B Johnston Memorial Hospital 40, 44, 51, 55, 100, 168
Gilmour, Mary 33
Goldmark Report 67–70, 84
Goode, Dr. 23, 84
Goodrich, Annie 36, 68
Goodrich, Frances 15
Grace Hospital NC 40, 42, 51, 54, 61, 168

Granny Banks 15–16, 134
Granny Midwives 4, 12–13, 112–115, 119, 134, 173
Greenville Sanitarium, Training School for Nurses 51
Greenwood, Mary 32
Guthrie Hospital 41, 46
Gwinn, Gladys 147

Hampton, Isabel 32–33, 35, 54, 72
Hancock, Glory 154–156
Harbin, Dr. R.M. 58
Harbin, Dr. W.P. 58
Harbin Hospital 30, 40, 43, 58–59
Hatfield, Henry 41, 47, 146
Healing Springs 22
Heim, Dr. Harlan 132–133
Henry Street Settlement 92, 94, 97, 106, 116
Higginbotham, Phyllis 139–141
Highland Hospital Asheville 50, 54, 86, 90
Highlands and Islands Medical Nursing Service 118, 125
Highlands Sanitarium, Chattanooga 28, 40, 44, 83–84, 156
Hindman Settlement School; 97, 130
Hinton Hospital, Hinton 46, 52, 56
Hobson, Archie 85–86, 88
Hodge, Lulu 64
Hoffman Hospital, Keyser 41, 47
Holman, Lydia 6, 95–98, 105–109
home remedies 61, 113
Honaker, Lou Willa 61
hookworm 138–139
Hot Springs 23
Howard Henderson Hospital Training School for Nurses 51, 55, 86
Huhn, Lula Mae 86
Huntington General Hospital 41, 46
Huntington Memorial Hospital 52, 57, 169
Hwang Hien Hospital China 156–157
Hyden Center 121–122, 124

Illinois Training School, Chicago 36

Jarvis, Amanda 64
Jefferson Hospital Roanoke 41, 45, 51, 55, 168
Jenkins, Geneva 157–158, 160–161
Jenkins, Ressa 157–158

Index

Jessie Preston Draper Center (Beech Fork Clinic) 121–122, 133
Johns Hopkins Hospital 32, 35–36, 64, 109
Johnston, Geroge Ben Memorial Hospital 40, 44, 47, 51, 55, 64–66, 100, 168

Kentucky Committee for Mothers and Babies 119, 121, 123
Kentucky Mountain Mission 131
Kessler-Hatfield Hospital 41, 47
Kings Daughters Hospital 41, 47
Knoxville General Hospital 47, 51, 55, 64, 76–77, 79–81, 85–86, 100, 103–104, 157, 164, 168, 170
Knoxville Private Hospital 40
Korean War 164–165

Laird Memorial Hospital Montgomery 53, 57, 169
Lakin State Hospital for the Colored Insane 87
Landrum and Litchfield of Abingdon 19
Lawler, Elsie 36
Lester, Betty 128
Lester, Jean 100
Lincoln Memorial Hospital 76, 82, 104
Lincoln Memorial University 75
Lobenstine Clinic 129
Logan Hospital 41, 47
Los Animas Hospital 152
Lounsberry, Harriet
Lowe, Agnes 169–171

Mackenzie, Sir Leslie 118, 125–126
MacKinnon, Ann 126
Madstones 19
Marsh, Ellen 133
Martinsburg Hospital 41, 47
Mason Hospital 41, 45
Massachusetts General Hospital, Boston 25
Massengill, Zella 86
Mayo, Dr. William 85
McBride, Grace 83–84, 156–157
McClung Hospital 41, 47
McDaniels, Grace 110
McElree's Wine of Cardui 20–22
McKean, Eva Ruth 110, 149
McKechnie, Mary 32
McKendree Hospital 41, 45, 52, 56, 146–148

McKendree Hospital (Miners Hospital #2) 41, 47, 53, 57, 146–148
McMillan, Helena 33
McMillan Hospital, Charleston 41, 45, 52, 56, 169
medical training 11–12, 14
medicine shows 20, 22, 188
Memorial Hospital, Johnson City 63, 64, 70–71, 82, 93
Memorial Hospital, Princeton 41
Memphis Training School for Nurses 151
Meriwether Hospital, Asheville 40, 43
Metropolitan Life Insurance 91–94, 99
midwifery 112–113, 115–116, 118, 121, 127–129, 133
military nursing 150–167
miners and medicine 147
Miners' Hospital 1 (Welch) 42, 47, 53, 57, 68, 109, 146
Miners' Hospital 2 (McKendree) 41, 47, 53, 57, 146–148
Miners' Hospital 3 (Fairmont) 41, 46, 52, 56, 66–67, 146–147, 169
missions and settlement schools 129–130, 139
Mitchell County, NC 6, 105–109
Moore, Frances 141
moral therapy 87
Mountain Home Veterans' Hospital 63, 170–171
Mountain Sanitarium and Hospital, Fletcher 51, 54
Mountain State Hospital, Charleston 52
Murphy, Dr. Patrick 87–89

National League of Nursing Education (NLNE) 29–33, 35–38, 50, 53, 57–58, 79, 100, 144–145
New York City Training School 91
New York Hospital 32, 91
New York Training School 33
Newell & Newell Sanitarium 40, 44, 51, 54
Nightingale, Florence 4, 24–25, 29–32, 71, 83, 91, 97, 150, 154, 173
NLNE Accreditation 29, 39, 50, 53–54
Normal Institute Hospital, Knoxville 40, 44
North Korea 165–166
Norton, Patty 111, 166
Noyes, Clara 33, 97, 101

191

Index

nurse anesthetists 81, 84, 86
Nurse Practice Act 73
Nurses' Associated Alumnae 71, 73
nursing education 24, 25, 27–41, 48–51, 53, 57–59, 61, 63, 65, 67–71, 73–74, 77–79, 81, 83–84, 86, 90, 100, 144–145, 150, 167
Nutting, Adelaide 33–34, 36, 48, 68

Oak Knoll Naval Hospital 170
Oak Ridge Hospital 170

Packard, Dr. George 15–16, 134–135, 154
Paine, Maggie 172
Paine, Terri 172
Paintsville General Hospital 40, 43, 60
Palmer, Sophia 32, 72
Parker Budd Clinic 51, 55
patent medicines 19, 21
Paulus, Jeanette 77–79
Peacock, Gladys 55, 122–123
Peplau, Hildegard 90
Pi Beta Phi 139, 141–142
polio epidemic 99–100, 142
Presbyterian Church Board of Home Missions 15, 134–135, 137, 154
Presbyterian Hospital, New York 33, 155
Protestant Episcopal Hospital, Philadelphia 79, 100–101
public health nurse 68, 92, 98, 101–102, 110–111, 133, 135, 152, 154
Puckett, Orlean 113–114

Qualla Boundary 110, 164, 169

railroad and Coal Mining 142, 145–146
Raleigh General Hospital, Beckley 52, 56, 169
Rankin, Mary 137–138
Red Bird 121, 131–133
Red Cross Public Health Nursing 91, 94–96, 99, 135–136, 154
Red Cross Town and Country Nursing Services 104
Reed Yellow Fever Board 152
Reid, Mrs. Whitelaw 95
Rice, Lydia 131–133
Rice, Mamie 65
Riddle, Mary 36
Riverside Hospital 40, 44

Roanoke Hospital 29, 41, 44–45, 50, 55, 169
Robertson, Katy 44, 56–57, 65
Rockefeller Foundation 67
Rockstroh, Edna 118, 121–122, 126

Sacred Heart Hospital 41, 47
St. Francis Hospital, Charleston 41, 45, 56, 169
St. Luke's Hospital, Bluefield 41, 45, 52, 56
St. Luke's Hospital, New Bedford, Massachusetts 33
St. Mary's, Clarksburg 52, 56, 169
St. Mary's Hospital, Huntington 41, 46, 53, 57, 169
Schiff, Jacob 94–95
Sheltering Arms Hospital 41, 46
Shenandoah Hospital 41, 45
Sheppard Towner Act 114–115
Singleton, Lena 64
Smith, Madge 144
Smith, Marie 64
Southwestern Virginia Mental Health Institute 87
Spanish American War 150–153, 174
Sprague, Lena 87, 89
SS Red Cross Hospital Ship 154
standard curriculum 36–37, 39, 48–49
State Boards of Nurse Examiners 39, 43
State Hospital for the Insane (Broughton) 85, 87–88
Sternberg 153, 158–159
Stewart, Isabel 36, 128
Stonega Coke and Coal Company 149
suffrage movement 59, 104
Sutliffe, Irene 32
Swartz, Vesta 64, 70–71

Takoma Hospital Training school for Nurses 51, 55
Teachers College 34, 36, 55, 90, 95, 98, 104, 118, 123, 128, 138
Tennessee Medical College 61, 75, 77
Tennessee State Board of Nurse Examiners (1922) 50–51, 79–80
Thedford's Black Draught 22
thrush 13, 18
Town and Country Nursing Service 95, 104
trachoma 111, 130
Tracy, Susan 36

Index

traditional healers 5, 11, 143, 146
Trans-Allegheny Lunatic Asylum 87
Trigg, Mary 80, 103–105

United Methodist Church 131
United States Cadet Nurse Corps 166–172
United States Public Health Service 60, 101, 167
University Hospital 32, 36, 84

Vardy, TN 137–138
visiting nursing 91–92, 94, 98–99, 103, 106, 109, 130

Wald, Lillian 68, 91–92, 94–96, 98, 116
Welch, Dr. William 68, 109

Welch Hospital (MH# 1) 42, 47, 53, 57
Wendover 121–122
West Ellis Hospital, Chattanooga 40, 44
Western North Carolina Insane Asylum 87
Wheeler, Mary 36
White, Lillian 26, 34–35, 77, 79–80, 100–101
White Rock Hospital 102, 133, 136, 154
Whiteside, Dr. Margaret 134
Willeford, Mary B 122–123, 134
Winslow, CEA 68, 126
World War I 63, 101, 135, 139, 152–157
World War II 157–158, 162, 166
Wytheville, Virginia 99–100

Yale University 69

www.ingramcontent.com/pod-product-compliance
Ingram Content Group UK Ltd.
Pitfield, Milton Keynes, MK11 3LW, UK
UKHW042009140426
5217IPUK00015B/1077